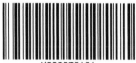

Smart Aging

Smart Aging

TAKING CHARGE OF YOUR
PHYSICAL AND EMOTIONAL HEALTH

Harriet Hodgson

(1999)

(1999)

John Wiley & Sons, Inc.

New York • Chichester • Weinheim • Brisbane • Singapore • Toronto

ISBN: 0-471-34797-3

Printed in the United States of America

10   9   8   7   6   5   4   3   2   · 1

Contents

Preface

We have all heard negative comments about aging. "Getting old is awful." "There's nothing good about aging." "Don't ever get old; I hate it." These kinds of comments reveal our society's fear of aging. You may have your own personal fears as well.

The fear of aging isn't limited to the over-50 folks. Teens worry about getting old and having wrinkled faces and gray hair. "Thirty somethings" are having their bodies sculpted (a nice word for liposuction), collagen injections, and various kinds of plastic surgery. The middle-aged and elderly are having multiple face lifts.

Savvy manufacturers are using the fear of aging to sell vitamins, hand lotion, cosmetics, toothpaste, candy bars, new cars, and a parade of other products. Some of us are so preoccupied with aging we miss the day we are living. This is more than a tragic waste of time, it discounts medical research.

Thanks to lower infant mortality, sanitation guidelines, better nutrition, and other advances in medicine our lives have been prolonged. We can look better and feel better longer. In fact, studies suggest we have some control over how long we live.

New definitions of aging have emerged from the research: young-old, middle-old (or middlescence), and old-old. Instead of sitting on the porch, seniors are running marathons, raising grandchildren, volunteering in schools, taking computer courses, launching new businesses, and traveling the globe, to name a few activities.

Yet some continue to generalize about older people and think anyone over 50 has squash rot; our brains have turned to mush. This is insulting and demeaning, as I learned at a local shopping mall.

I was in a hurry, so I bought a sweater without trying it on. The sweater didn't fit and I returned it the next day. "I'd like to make an even exchange," I told the sales associate. "This sweater is too small. I'll get a larger one."

When I laid the sweaters on the counter the sales associate looked me over quickly. "This is the sweater you brought in," she said slowly, enunciating each word. "And this is the sweater you want to take home." She pointed to each sweater as she spoke to me.

Her patronizing manner rendered me speechless. I wanted to shout, "And this is my fist in your face!" The experience was doubly painful because the sales associate was a woman. Aren't women supposed to stick together? I wondered why she thought I was demented.

Apparently the sales associate, who was in her early 20s, had not faced her own aging. Aging is inevitable and it happens to everyone. Getting older doesn't mean we are confused and purposeless. Just the opposite may be true and we may be more purposeful about life.

I am in my 60s now, plugging along with a writing career, volunteering in my community, savoring the joys of grandparenting, and more in love with my husband than ever. We recently celebrated our 41st wedding anniversary. For me, this is a rich and satisfying time of life.

In her book, *Wouldn't Take Nothing for My Journey Now*,

Maya Angelou has a chapter called "Passports to Understanding." This is a good description of the aging process. For the longer we live the more we understand life. Indeed, I think understanding is the quest.

How we approach aging has a lot to do with how we plan our lives.

Due to the tragedy and pain I have experienced I am excited to be alive. Not everyone feels as I do and, frankly, I am sick of the whining. The idea for this book came to me in the grocery store after hearing two couples discuss aging. Their conversation was an endless list of complaints.

I drove home, put the groceries away, and took out my grocery list. On the back of the list I jotted down some of the positives of aging. Because of my age:

- I know who I am.
- I know what I can do.
- I have an idea of what I can't do.
- I take better care of myself.
- I take credit for what I have done.
- I accept challenges.
- I try to do the right thing.
- I am more committed to my family and others.

"It's a book," I muttered to myself. A book about aging was a logical step after writing two books on Alzheimer's disease, which detail my mother's dementia. During the last year of her life I was caught in a terrible paradox, a cruel and painful twist of fate.

As my mother's life was ending, mine seemed to be starting over again, and I felt reborn. I still feel this way. Each morning I awaken with a sense of wonder and purpose. The purpose of this book is to give you a balanced view of aging.

Before I did any writing I checked other books in print. Some of the titles make outrageous claims that defy medical research. It seems we don't want to face the truth about aging and are looking for the miracle of the week. The miracle is in view and it is life.

This book takes you from thoughts about aging to physical changes, to planning for the future. In researching the book I used the Medline database, medical newsletters, newspaper and magazine articles, and personal interviews. I also conducted a random survey, called "How Do You Feel About Aging?"

There were five questions on the form:

1. What are some good things about aging?

2. What are some bad things about aging?

3. What activities do you enjoy?

4. Occupation?

5. Age?

I surveyed community contacts and people who used our local Senior Citizens Center. The center made a special box for the forms and displayed it by the entrance. To my surprise, the response from the center was poor. "They don't want to think about aging," the secretary said ruefully, "and they sure don't like to fill out forms!"

Four people put blank survey forms in the box. Was this a protest? Did their lives seem blank? Were these people suffering from dementia? I have no way of knowing. Although my survey was small, a total of 50 respondents, it gave me many helpful insights.

Some responses are touching, others are hilarious. A 71-year-old woman wrote, "Kids are gone, dog died, now we are free." You may feel the same way. But studies show that many of us fail to plan for aging. We think we have lots of time and planning is too much trouble.

If we are going to have the freedom we envision we must plan our future. No matter how old you are, every adult needs an aging plan. Start your plan now. This book is packed with tips and all of them are based on research.

I have included personal stories to make the research real to you. Headings make the book easy to use and each chapter ends with "Smart Aging Tips," a summary of the points discussed. Page through the book and resource list before you start reading.

Yes, problems come with aging, but there are many advantages as well. Let us find the courage to savor every moment—the joy, the pain, the challenges, the wonder—of this amazing journey of life. These days will not come again.

(2021 OCTOBER)

1

Aging as a State of Mind

When I was growing up, 50-year-olds were considered elderly. They weren't expected to do much, other than care for children, cook hearty meals, and sit on the porch. The seeds for our ideas about aging are planted in childhood, although we may not see the fruits for years.

My mother died on November 12, 1997, just before the holidays, and all of my preparations were tinged with sadness. The holidays were bittersweet. I kept thinking about Mom, staring at her photograph and expecting her to talk to me. Sometimes I thought I heard her laugh.

My brother called me right after Mom died. I asked him how he was doing. "Well, I've had better weeks," he said, pausing for a moment. "I used to have people running interference for me. Now I'm out in front."

His sports analogy is a good one. I, too, feel like I'm out in front. My mother's death provoked a flood of childhood memories. I thought about the simple views my parents instilled in me. Be honest. Work hard. Do your best. Each of my parents gave me different emotional gifts and I use them all.

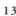

Family Influence

My father was a second generation American. His childhood ended abruptly when his father was killed in a car accident. The only healthy son in an impoverished family, Dad was forced to quit school in the eighth grade and work to support the family. He started out as a messenger boy and eventually became a paint salesman. Despite a limited education, Dad was a brilliant man, and he was always trying out new formulas in the basement. At our house Dad's messy, dented, paint-dripped workbench (next to the furnace) was sacred. Failure didn't stop Dad and if an experiment didn't work he tried it again. And again. His persistence led to the development of new products.

I am a lot like my father.

Also a second generation American, my mother quit school in the 11th grade. She worked as a secretary in New York's famous garment district and occasionally modeled stockings. The middle child in a family of five children, Mom had a witty, adaptive, and practical personality. Her approach to life is revealed in a story she told me.

It seems a church friend stopped by to ask Mom's advice. "She told me such a tale of woe," Mom recalled. "Unfaithful husband. Money problems. Kids in trouble."

"What did you say?" I asked.

"I told her to get over it!" she exclaimed.

Mom's retort has become a family joke, and my husband and I use it often. Every time we say it we laugh. But the philosophy behind the reply wasn't a joke. Despite a difficult, at times harsh life, Mom continued to adapt.

I am a lot like my mother.

Become aware of your family's influence on your ideas about aging. You may agree with these ideas or challenge them; the choice is yours. Family influence can be a starting point for personal growth. Add research findings to this starting point and you will have a better understanding of your ideas about aging.

The crucial question is whether the aging brain can continue to learn. Or to put it another way, can the brain continue to store and retrieve data? The answer to this question affects everyone. Much has been learned about the brain in the last few years, although many of its workings remain a mystery.

Memory

Thanks to Magnetic Resonance Imaging, or MRI, we can now see the human brain. Even more amazing, we can see the brain at work. Research is changing our ideas about brain function. Mary Carman, PhD, conducted a longitudinal study of aging and reported the results in her study, "The Psychology of Normal Aging."

Carman found that aging alters the brain's ability to function efficiently. Some of the changes:

- Aging people experience a decline in short-term memory (20 seconds or less)
- Some aging people (not all) experience a decline in logical thinking after age 70
- Some aging people (not all) experience a decline in verbal ability after age 70
- Every age group has its "top performers"

I think variation is the encouraging news here. Being in your 50s, 60s, and 70s doesn't mean your mind is going to give out. You may continue to lead a satisfying life. However, you may have more grief experiences along the way.

Carman also found that grief alters our ability to learn. Time is supposed to heal all wounds, according to an old adage, and Carman tells us how much time. "Research suggests that it requires approximately 18 months to 2 years for the physiological systems to return to baseline following a grief incident."

It's easy to understand this concept intellectually and hard to understand it emotionally. As we get older more loved ones and friends die. Like sand tracked in from the beach, grief works its way into every nook and cranny of our lives. We think we have swept up all of the sand—the grief—and then it reappears.

A neighbor of mine had five relatives die in three months. Her life became nothing more than grief. Thank goodness she was wise enough to get professional help.

Carman's research reminds us to be kind to ourselves. We can give ourselves permission to go slowly, to progress one day and regress the next. If we're a little forgetful in the process, so be it. All of us forget things at one time or another. However, some of us can't stop complaining about our memory problems.

Memory Complaints

We may lose our car keys, or even our cars. After our daughter was hospitalized due to injuries sustained in a near-fatal car crash, I couldn't remember where I parked the car. To make matters worse, my car was silver, and there were dozens of silver cars in the hospital lot. It took me a half hour to find my car and I was angry at myself.

Several weeks later I was even angrier. I was writing a book (well into the middle of it) and realized I couldn't recall simple words. Although I could see the shapes of the words in my mind, I couldn't remember the words themselves. The next morning the words would pop into my mind.

Stress had short-circuited my mind's retrieval system.

Once I knew our daughter was on the road to recovery my memory returned to normal. It took several months, though, and the process was painful. All the while, I kept wondering if my memory would fail again.

Tuomo Hännien, MA, and his colleagues examined memory complaints in aging people in Kuopio, Finland, chosen because of its elderly population. Their results are detailed in the study, "Subjective Memory Complaints and Personality Traits in Normal Elderly Subjects."

Their study examines the relationship between memory complaints and actual function.

A large group of randomly selected participants started out in the study. This group was whittled down to two matched groups. Each participant was given a memory complaint questionnaire about ordinary events, such as losing car keys, forgetting grocery lists, and other memory problems.

The participants were also given the Minnesota Multiphasic Personality Inventory (MMPI) and a geriatric depression test. When the test results were evaluated the subjects' complaints didn't match their performance. In short, the people who complained the most were chronic complainers.

"The high scores on these MMPI scales indicate stronger tendencies toward somatic complaining, anxiety about physical health, and inferior feelings about personal competence and capabilities," the researchers explain.

Learn to tell the difference between real and imaginary memory complaints. Contact your doctor if you can't tell the difference. Also become aware of the influence of your personality upon aging. You may be an extrovert, the kind of person who always finds something to laugh about, or you may be wary of life.

Personality

Personality is defined within a framework of culture and life experience. For example, I am originally from Long Island, New York, and have an Eastern sense of humor. Midwesterners don't always understand my humor and look at me oddly. I don't always understand Scandinavian humor and the "Ole and Lena" jokes that are popular in Minnesota.

Researcher Mary Carman thinks personality remains fairly constant over time. Some of my friends have personalities similar to mine, whereas others are quite different. Recently a friend and I met for lunch. Another friend joined us to chat. We had so much news to share that we all talked at once.

In fifteen minutes we covered aging, grandchildren, and menopause. The man at the next table was so fascinated by our conversation he kept turning around to peek at us. His behavior made him part of our group and Laura bid him good-bye when she left.

"I've never heard anything like this," he laughed. "It's been fun."

I turned around and asked, "So how's the family?" He laughed even harder. Since I hadn't ordered my food yet, I asked the man what he was eating.

"It's the soup and sandwich combo," he replied. "Chicken soup, real spicy, but good." He moved aside so I could get a better view of his lunch. "Want a taste? Here, I have a clean spoon."

"No thanks," I said. "I think I'll avoid the spicy stuff and order something else."

Lunch was pure serendipity. I don't think any of this would have happened if my friends and I didn't have similar personalities. We're outgoing, quick to laugh, interested in art and antiques. Personality influences our response to change. Draw upon your personality strengths as you grow older.

Coping with Change

Change is like the wind, altering direction and force without warning. Just when we think we know how to cope with change it catches us off guard. We must polish our coping skills, find new ways of coping, or do both.

Renee Solomon, DSW, and Monte Peterson, MD, examine

the human responses to change in their study, "Successful Aging: How to Help Your Patients Cope With Change." The researchers think aging people can lead quality lives if they learn to:

- Cope with the physical/emotional stress of aging
- Retain some control over their personal lives
- Stay connected with family members and friends
- See their lives as meaningful

I would add "develop new interests" to their list. Many of the retired people I know have taken up new hobbies, such as golf. One of my friends moved to the Southwest and became fascinated with local history. Sometimes though, no matter how adaptive we may be, our coping batteries run down.

Where do we turn? Solomon and Peterson say we can turn to community resources. They also advise us to be flexible and find meaningful ways to spend our time.

People are different, and what is meaningful to you may seem meaningless to me. Still, we can be open to new experiences. "The ability to view change as meaningful to one's life is another key to successful aging," the researchers write. You may find yourself restructuring your life.

I think we also need something to anticipate. It doesn't have to be a big thing, it can be a little thing, such as Halloween. The holiday is as exciting for me as it is for our twin grandchildren (one boy, one girl) because their excitement is contagious. "You give us more because you know us. Right, Grandma?" they ask.

(Stress)

Today's stress differs from the stress of the past, according to Marion Zucker Goldstein, MD, and Cathy Ann Perkins, MD. They pinpoint some of the differences in their study, "Mental Health and the Aging Woman." In past years these things were normal for women:

- ■ Few life choices (I could be a teacher or a nurse.)
- ■ Sex discrimination (Remember, women had to demonstrate and lobby for the right to vote.)
- ■ Biased legislation, education, and health care
- ■ Living alone (or being the spinster of the family)
- ■ Lack of support when caring for children/parents
- ■ Widowhood with a low chance of remarriage

While these factors haven't disappeared entirely, women's lives are improving. Society is more aware of the psychological differences between the sexes. As the researchers note, "Women define their identity through relationships of intimacy and care, whereas power and separation secure men's identity." Aging women are becoming more powerful in our country. Women 65 years old and older are the fastest growing segment of our society. This statistical shift is having a profound effect on the public's perception of aging.

An increasing number of stock market investors are women. According to the Home Business Administration, 300,000 women start home businesses each year. Starting a new business is stressful for anyone, male or female. Like other home-based workers, I have found that some people don't validate my efforts. They think I am "putzing." In their minds, a gray-haired grandmother can't possibly be a viable member of the workforce. Nothing changes their minds, not even books with my name on the cover. I find this narrow viewpoint rather stressful.

Learning to identify the stressors takes lots of practice. Stressors change with the circumstances. To make myself more aware of the stressors in my life I keep a list on a small pad. If I can learn to spot stressors, you can too.

When you feel yourself getting anxious, put the brakes on, and take care of yourself. I eliminate the minor stressors first and work up to the major ones. You may follow this pattern or work in reverse. Figure out what works best for you.

Loss and Loneliness

Aging people go through a series of losses. We have physical losses, such as the loss of agility. We have emotional losses, such as the death of a cherished pet. Our losses add up over time. Certainly, the loss of a spouse can drastically alter our view of life.

A widow refused to complete the aging survey because her spouse had died. "You see things differently when you've lost a husband," she explained. "My responses wouldn't help you. Ask someone else."

After a spouse dies some people feel their lives are over, or at the very least, a dark void. Loneliness is a powerful emotion. After moving 15 or 16 times (I lost track) I understand the power of loneliness. Adjusting to a new community takes time, discipline, and old-fashioned hard work.

You may feel alone in your own hometown. When my dearest friend moved away, my main support system also moved away. I was overcome with loneliness. I knew social activity was the solution, but loneliness made me withdraw into myself even more.

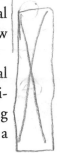

Finally I forced myself to call friends. It took me several months to find my social skills, dust them off, and reactivate them. Remember that loneliness isn't the same as being alone. You can feel alone in a noisy football stadium or a theater packed to capacity.

Because my husband is a health professional I have spent a lot of time alone. Over the years I have learned how to rely on myself, trust my judgment, and be content with my own company. I cope with loneliness by making a loneliness plan. If my husband is going to be out of town I make a list of possible activities. I keep the list in my kitchen junk

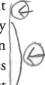

drawer, along with brochures and newspaper ads. The plan calls for contact with our grown children, twin grandchildren, and friends. However, I only go out at night if I am with a group.

I think the violence in our society adds to the loneliness we feel. We used to leave our houses and cars unlocked. Now we have security devices on our cars, deadbolt locks on our doors, and mace cans in our pockets. While these self-protection measures are comforting, they are also alarming.

Society seems to be forcing us into cocoons of loneliness. With notable exceptions, the young and the old tend to lead separate lives in America. I have seen kids cross the street to avoid contact with older people. We need to link the generations together, not go our separate ways.

The "Moany-Groanies"

Aches and pains go along with aging. Our feet hurt from walking on them all these years. High school sports injuries may start to act up again. It takes us longer to do things. These kinds of ailments may lead us to the doctor and he or she may prescribe medicine for us.

Many aging people have the "moany-groanies," a litany of ailments and medications they constantly recount for others. The day after my father died my husband and I flew to Long Island to attend his funeral. Relatives had gathered at our home to mourn my father's passing.

They brought the moany-groanies with them. Pills were the main topic of conversation at meal time: the number of pills, what they were for, and when they were taken. Each relative took out his or her pills and put them on the table. One by one, they took the pills. I expected to hear about their bowel movements at any minute.

Please understand that I sympathize with my relatives' health problems, but I think they could have picked a better time to discuss them. As more loved ones and friends die,

Smart Aging

however, we have fewer people to talk with, to test and validate our ideas. I didn't realize this until my widowed mother moved to Florida.

During my visits I noticed that Mom shared very personal information with strangers. Why was she doing this? Although her sister lived in the same city, she lived on the other side of town, and Mom rarely saw her. Mom was so starved for companionship that she shared her thoughts with neighbors, cashiers, mail carriers, bank tellers— anyone who would listen. HAIRDRESSER

Experts say depression is on the rise in our country. I think lack of companionship may be one reason for this.

Let's take a look at some of the current depression research. As you read the next section remember that depression strikes people of all ages.

Depression in the Aging

According to American Psychiatric Association reports, 40 to 50 million people in America have the symptoms of mental illness each year. Depression is the most common form of mental illness. If we live long enough, the time comes when we need help with the activities of daily living: bathing, dressing, cooking, shopping. This is depressing, to say the least.

Some experts think depression is a normal part of the aging process.

Martha Livingston Bruce, PhD, MPH, and her associates examined depression and reported their findings in a study called "The Impact of Depressive Symptomatology on Physical Disability: MacArthur Studies of Successful Aging." After looking at earlier data and conducting follow-up interviews, the researchers say depression is not a normal part of aging.

What's more, they say depression is a "potentially preventable condition." This is good news. Unfortunately, aging people may hide their depression because they think it will go away by itself or consider it a character flaw. Disease may also mask the symptoms of depression. So doctors are screening their patients more carefully for it.

Barry Lebowitz, PhD, and his colleagues spotlight depression in their study, "Diagnosis and Treatment of Depression in Late Life." The researchers think the evidence for long-term treatment of depression is mounting. "Older patients with recurrent depression may need antidepressant treatment indefinitely to remain well."

New drugs have been developed to treat depression. With the right drugs and the right dosage, depressed patients have shown dramatic improvement. But the statistics on mental illness keep going up and nobody seems to know why. Aging people who are mentally ill want to retain some control over their lives. Is this goal realistic?

Kristine Tower, MSW, LCSW, discusses the issue in her study, "Consumer-Centered Social Work Practice: Restoring Client Self-Determination." She attributes the changing national policies and services to the "revival of consumer activity." Groups for the mentally ill, special clubs and clubhouses, and better transportation services have come from this revival.

Tower says social workers, who are both facilitators and role models, have helped to spark these changes. "They [social workers] can encourage their clients to take purposeful action to improve their condition through self-advocacy and organizations with peers."

Despite this and other kinds of self-advocacy, our society doesn't understand mental illness very well. Mental illness is often regarded as something to fear. Myths about mental illness still persist. An article in the Menninger Perspective, "Myths About Mental Illness," details some common myths.

MYTH 1: Average people aren't affected by mental illness.

MYTH 2: All mentally ill people are dangerous.

MYTH 3: Young children don't get mental illness.

MYTH 4: Seeing a mental health professional is a sign of weakness.

MYTH 5: Mentally ill people don't recover.

Every one of these myths is false. What is true, however, is that some aging people are mentally ill. Their illness may be caused by crisis, changes in brain chemistry, medication intolerance, stroke damage, Alzheimer's disease, or other forms of dementia.

Mental illness distorts the person's view of the world in much the same way as wearing the wrong glasses distorts vision. Everything looks blurry and out of focus. Dr. Donald Rosen, head of the Menninger Professionals in Crisis program, thinks many mental illnesses are a one-time thing and says, "Once treated, they never recur; there is complete recovery."

Rosen thinks we need mental health professionals as much as we need medical health professionals. Early intervention leads to a better outcome, according to Rosen. See your doctor if you think you are depressed. Be prepared to answer questions about the medicine you are taking because medicine can alter thinking.

Medication and the Mind

People have harmed themselves by mixing drugs, taking too many drugs, and taking them too long. A *New York Times* News Service article, "Patients Over 60 Are Cautioned on Painkillers," summarizes a survey of people age 59 and older who were taking painkillers. Nearly three-quarters of the people took the prescription or over-the-counter medicine longer than prescribed. This is a dangerous practice, especially if the painkillers are mixed with alcohol. Certainly, an impaired mind isn't a rational mind.

Studies such as this one emphasize the need for reading labels carefully. I carry a flexible plastic magnifying lens (the size of a bookmark) in my purse. Bookstores used to carry the lenses, but they are becoming scarce. Other inexpensive magnifying glasses are available, however.

Doctors also recommend keeping a medication diary. It's a good way to track what you are taking and when you take it. Don't fall for the "If one pill is good more must be better" theory. Above all, don't believe all of the advertising claims you hear. You need to know what you are putting into your body.

Remember that older people tolerate medicine differently than younger people. Drug interactions may also cause health problems. Call your doctor if you have any questions about the medicine you are taking.

Sense of Self

Before I became a writer I taught preschool, kindergarten, and teacher certification workshops. Usually I did a unit with the children called "This is Me." The children made self-portraits, shared family photos, cut out pictures of their favorite foods, discussed their feelings, and dictated stories to me about themselves.

I have been thinking about the unit because my sense of self has changed. A few years ago I wasn't a grandmother. Time has expanded my sense of self and, much as I hate to admit it, my waistline. I have a strong sense of self and it boils down to these basics:

- These are my talents.
- This is my training.
- This is what I do.
- This is my experience.
- These are my values.
- These are my goals.

Goals are important in our lives, no matter how old we are, and we need to work toward them. You may work toward your goals with studied seriousness or childlike fun. Being goal-oriented doesn't mean you eliminate surprise from your life.

Surprising Ourselves

I surprised myself when I hiked up the Inca Trail above Machu Picchu, Peru. Three months before the trip I started training on the stationary bike. My training paid off. I had no problem with the 7,000 foot altitude or the additional climb up the mountain toward the Inca Gate, a dark gray silhouette against a light gray sky. The trail was my problem.

It started as a wide dirt road, narrowed to a foot-wide path, and finally became a rock ledge suspended in air. I have a fear of heights and when I saw the ledge I gulped. Recent eye surgery for a detaching retina fueled my fear. There was little vegetation to break my fall, and I pictured myself rolling down the mountain side to the valley floor far below me.

I could see the miniature train station and miniature people walking about. Good grief, I could roll into the station along with the train. Suddenly I burst into tears. "People with a fear of heights shouldn't be doing this," I cried.

My husband, who always respects my feelings, hugged me and said we should go back. As we started our descent he remembered his jacket, left behind on the trail when he stopped to take a picture. While he went to retrieve his jacket, I sat down and waited for him. (Actually, I was clinging to a rock.)

I tried not to think about the altitude or an article I had read about bandits on the Inca Trail. Above me, I heard people speaking in Spanish, and two scruffy looking men appeared. They were wearing huge backpacks and carrying walking sticks. One reached for something behind his back.

"Oh, oh, this is it," I thought to myself. "He is going to rob me." But he didn't rob me, he offered me his water bottle.

"Agua, señora?" he asked.

"No, gracias," I replied.

He asked me some questions and, realizing I understood little Spanish, asked "OK?" There was genuine concern in his face.

"Si, gracias," I answered.

Other hikers passed me on the trail and they were equally as kind. A few minutes later my husband returned and we resumed our descent. Going down the trail was harder than going up, and I held onto every rock, branch, and twig I could find. Yet I was proud of myself. I had trained successfully, hiked at high altitude, and nearly reached the Inca Gate. A few tears were nothing in comparison to these accomplishments.

You may surprise yourself by running for office, heading a neighborhood watch, or taking up a new hobby. Age doesn't cancel out the wonder of life and some of us have a renewed sense of spirituality. How you apply this spirituality to life is a personal decision.

Spirituality

Many of us seek spiritual help only in times of crisis.

Jacqueline Ruth Mickley, PhD, RN, and other researchers review the history of religion in a study called, "Religion and Adult Mental Health: State of the Science in Nursing." They think spirituality impacts health by:

- Helping us to lead healthy lives
- Fostering social concern/cohesiveness
- Easing stress (through prayer)
- Helping us to find meaning in our lives
- Connecting us to an "ultimate another"

The researchers think spirituality is a necessity of life.
They write, "A wide range of studies has shown that individuals who demonstrate high levels of intrinsic religiousness tend to have less depression, anxiety, and dysfunctional attention seeking, and high levels of ego strength, empathy, and integrated social behavior."

Watching my friends care for their spiritual selves has been interesting. One friend had converted to a different religion and returned to the religion of her childhood later in life. She sings in the choir and participates in many of the church's social events. Another friend, one of the most spiritual people I know, became an agnostic.

Spiritual beliefs come from the core of our being. I define my spirituality in simple terms: do no harm, do my best, be kind to others. Nature is a continuous source of spirituality for me.

Seeing the giant redwood trees in California made me feel like I was in the presence of God. The trees reached toward the sky like giant church spires and the branches sheltered me like a timbered roof. I can still see the trees in my mind, feel the rough bark, and hear the wind in the boughs.

As we grow older we need to stay in touch with our spiritual selves. More friends seem to be sharing their spiritual experiences with me. It doesn't matter that some of their spiritual views differ from mine. We are as aware of our spiritual aging as we are of physical aging. Maybe the two go hand in hand.

PAINTING

Talk About Aging

Growing older changed me from Miss, to Ms to Ma'am. I remember the day a gas station employee called me ma'am. For a brief time I mourned this change because it was a reflection of my age. (I got over it.) The things we say reveal our thoughts about aging.

English is a rich language, filled with adjectives to help us

to express our ideas. Our language is also filled with slang.
There are many slang words for aging people: *codger, coot,*
and *geezer* for men, *blue-haired old ladies, biddies,* and *gossips*
for women. Not only are these words unkind, they are communication blockers.

The questions we ask may also hinder communication.
My father-in-law, who is a handsome, intelligent, and
charismatic man, gave me some good advice. "When people
ask, 'How are you,' say 'Fine.' Don't complain." He makes a
good point. Most people don't want an answer to this question.

Plus, we make strangers feel uncomfortable if we share
too much with them. When we have gotten to know someone better, we may be more forthcoming. Any grandparent
knows that children are very forthcoming with their ideas.

"Grandma, are you old?" my granddaughter asked.

"Yes," I answered. "If I wasn't old I wouldn't be your
grandma." My granddaughter looked at me intently,
smiled, and kissed me on the cheek. I would not trade my
grandchildren for youth, for they have enriched my life in
ways I never imagined.

Author Ruth Harriet Jacobs writes about age in her
poem, "Don't Call Me a Young Woman," which is included
in her book, *Be An Outrageous Older Woman.* The poem
takes Jacobs from youth, to middle age, to old age. Jacobs
says the words "young woman" are insulting and reveal the
speaker's fear of aging.

According to Jacobs, age is a hard-won achievement, and
she considers her gray hair and wrinkles "badges of triumphant survival." Life tests us all in different ways. Your
triumphant survival may depend on whether or not you age
gracefully.

Graceful Aging

The word graceful has several definitions; one, according to Webster's, is elegance or beauty of form, manner, motion, or action and moral strength. All of these factors influence graceful aging, but there is more to it. Graceful aging is knowing when to be silent and when to speak up, when to advance and when to retreat, when to negotiate and when to take a stand.

In order to age gracefully you need a plan, or map. Your map may not be identical to mine, but it gives you something to go by. Even a roughly drawn map gives you a sense of direction. Add details to your map when you feel like it, and, when your map gets worn, make a new one.

Nobody can predict how many maps you will need in your lifetime. Although our destinations differ, aging is the route that gets us there. Graceful aging requires special courage, a quiet, steady, solid resolve we may draw upon all through life. Forging this courage takes time and is, by itself, a courageous act.

The final requirement of graceful aging is enjoyment.

In her memoir, *Any Given Day*, eighty-year-old Jessie Lee Brown Foveaux details her approach to life. "I realize that my happy days can come to an end anytime, so I shall just enjoy each day." I think this is sound advice.

This chapter has focused on some of the factors that shape your view of aging. While aging is something we do with others, it is really a solitary journey, a journey of body, mind, and spirit. These tips will help you find your way.

Smart Aging Tips

- Become aware of your family's influence on your ideas about aging.
- Learn to tell the difference between memory complaints and memory loss.
- Draw upon your personality strengths as you age.
- Learn how to cope with change.
- Identify the stressors in your life and do something about them.
- Make a loneliness plan.
- See your doctor if you think you are depressed.
- Read all prescription and nonprescription labels carefully.
- Retain your sense of self.
- Surprise yourself every once in a while.
- Find comfort and direction in spirituality.
- Talk positively about aging.
- Try to age gracefully.

2

Physical Aspects of Aging

"*Your book won't be* worth a plug nickel if you don't tell what aging does to the body," a friend declared. She is right. The effects of aging cannot be denied. Despite our different genes, environments, and lifestyles, aging is the one thing we have in common.

What does aging do to you? Pamela Maxson and her associates focus on the general effects of aging in their study, "Multidimensional Patterns of Aging: A Cluster-Analytic Approach," published in *Experimental Aging Research.* Aging is a complex series of processes, the researchers explain, and these processes shape our "trajectory of aging."

Building on data from a previous geriatric study in Gothenburg, Sweden, the researchers examine "five domains" of aging:

1. Physical health
2. Cognitive performance
3. Subjective well-being
4. Social contacts
5. Functional capacity

The researchers did a cluster analysis and a longitudinal analysis of data. They say one of the main features of this approach is that patterns emerge from the data, rather than preconceived groupings. Although the five domains don't cover every variation in aging, the results of the study are encouraging.

"Many of the subjects were in high-functioning groups, contradicting the widespread assumption that old age is primarily a time of general decrement," note the researchers.

In short, many of us will continue to live cogent, productive, and satisfying lives. Of course we will still encounter age-related problems; aches and pains come with the territory. So does a loss of height, which is common in aging people.

Height

Loss of height may be barely noticeable or obvious. During my last physical exam I was surprised to discover I had shrunk an inch. Despite fifteen years of hormone replacement therapy (HRT) and calcium supplements, I still had some height loss. How much shorter would I be without this therapy?

I didn't notice my loss of height because it happened slowly. The same thing could happen to you. If you are female, ask your doctor if you need a bone density test.

The test is usually done on women, but men may also need it.

Osteoporosis is another cause of height loss. The discs between the vertebrae may flatten out, causing the person to shrink. Kyphosis, or curving of the spine, is yet another cause. My loss of height didn't change my self-image, however, and I still think of myself as a tall person.

Weight

Aging people often gain weight. Although I didn't notice my loss of height, I was very aware of my weight gain. The point struck home every time I bought new clothes. Normal weight, that is, what is normal for you, depends on genetics, diet, and exercise. Hormones may also play a part.

According to Regina Casper of the Stanford University School of Medicine in California, "Hormone systems can be less responsive with advancing age." She discusses nutrition and weight gain in her study, "Nutrition and its Relationship to Aging." Although the National Academy of Sciences has issued daily food allowances for people ages 23 to 50 and people over 50, Casper says no standards exist for determining the caloric intake for aging people.

The National Academy of Science standards are broad ones, Casper adds, and don't take our personal differences into account. Then too, our nutritional needs vary according to our activity level. Someone who is doing manual labor needs more calories than someone who is sedentary, for example.

Being overweight is more common in aging people than being underweight. Where you carry your weight depends on your body type—apple or pear.

I am a pear, a very pleasant pear, I think, but a pear nevertheless. Experts say pear-shaped people have a lower risk of heart disease than apple-shaped people. "Fat deposition around the waist as reflected by a high ratio of waist to hip circumference is associated with greater health risk than fat deposition in the hips," writes Casper.

Researchers are working on ways to reduce fat deposits, largely through exercise and healthier eating.

Hormone replacement therapy (HRT) may also lead to weight gain. Fatty tissue is deposited in the breasts, fanny, thighs, and stomach. Women who have been on estrogen for many years develop an "estrogen tummy." Personally, I think HRT is a trade-off, and would rather have an estrogen tummy than brittle bones.

Eyes

Our eyes may not see as well as they did in the past. You may have floaters, dry eyes, depth perception problems, glare sensitivity, or become near-sighted or far-sighted. Thank goodness we live at a time when contact lenses, laser surgery, and lens implants are possible.

I attributed my early vision problems to fatigue. The fatigue excuse failed the day my husband met me at the San Francisco airport. Judging by his contour and walk, I thought the man coming toward me was my husband, and opened my arms to hug him. At the last second I realized he was a stranger.

The open-arms gesture is hard to change. Should I scratch my back? Should I shift my raincoat to the other arm? Should I reach for something? I grinned at the stranger and he grinned back because he knew what had happened. "Wrong man," I said sheepishly, and we laughed. A few weeks later I was wearing glasses.

Vision problems may contribute to highway accidents. Two researchers at the University of Kentucky, Nikiforos Stamatiadis and John Deacon, detail vision problems in their study, "Trends in Highway Safety: Effects of an Aging Population on Accident Propensity." They say the aging eye has problems with focusing, changing focus, depth perception, peripheral vision, and in some cases, color blindness.

Any one of these problems makes night driving difficult.

Cataracts may also obscure our vision. Allen Taylor and his colleagues look at the relationship between nutrition and the development of cataracts in their study, "Relations Among Aging, Antioxidant Status, and Cataract." Aging may cause the lenses in our eyes to become less flexible, they explain, a condition called "age-related cataract."

While it's too soon to say poor nutrition causes cataracts, the researchers think improving diet may delay onset. This may be achieved "with the aid of supplements once appropriate amounts of specifically beneficial nutrients are defined."

Your eyes may feel dryer as you get older. Buy a bottle of artificial tears if this has happened to you. I take them with me on trips because pressurized plane cabins dry out my eyes. Instead of carbonated beverages, I drink plain water to stay hydrated.

Prescription sunglasses are expensive, so I wear wraparound glasses over my regular glasses. You can find the wraparounds at discount stores and they come in several tints. I also have a pair of clip-on sunglasses that go over my regular glasses.

Ears

The world is a noisy place, filled with piercing background noise, transportation noise, and music played at damaging decibels. Noise pollution can damage our hearing. Loud appliances, such as vacuum cleaners, may also cause hearing damage.

Jay Pearson and his colleagues at the National Institute on Aging in Baltimore examine the causes of hearing loss in their study, "Gender Differences in a Longitudinal Study of Age-Associated Hearing Loss."

The purpose of the study was to describe hearing loss in terms of age and gender. A total of 1,097 people were in the study, 681 men and 416 women. Men and women were given continuous pure-tone hearing tests and pulsed pure-tone hearing tests at regular intervals. Some of the study findings:

- Hearing sensitivity in men declines significantly at age 20
- "After age 30, hearing sensitivity in women declines cross-sectionally at all frequencies."

- Men who are 30 years old and older have better hearing thresholds than women (at 500 Hz)
- More men have high-frequency loss than women
- "Among women, hearing levels worsen at all ages for 500 Hz."

The moral of this study is to get your hearing checked. Hearing loss isn't confined to the aging. Kids may also have hearing loss, especially if they play in a rock band or listen to loud music at home or in the car. Have your hearing checked if you are exposed to high noise levels over a sustained period of time. It's better to be safe than sorry.

You might want to carry earplugs with you. Buy several sets because the plugs get lost easily. I prefer the spongy ones made for professional crafters. They meet OSHA standards and protect you up to 28 decibels when used as directed. To insert the plugs, you roll them with clean hands to the smallest diameter. Insert the tapered end of the plug into your ear canal and hold it in place until expanded. The plugs are inexpensive and come three pairs to a package.

Tinnitus, a continuous pitch or ringing in the ears, may also be a problem for you. Of course there isn't any actual ringing; the ears are sending a false signal to the brain.

My father's tinnitus got worse when he was in his 50s. All day and all night, he heard ringing in his ears, and it drove him nuts. Dad was a volunteer fireman and the firehouse siren was almost the same pitch as his tinnitus. "Is that the siren?" he would ask. He must have asked me this question five times a week. Tinnitus put my father in a constant state of readiness. Sometimes it really was the siren, and Dad would grab his jacket and run down the street to the firehouse.

Annoying as it was, tinnitus didn't alter Dad's satisfaction in being a volunteer fireman. Usually people who have tinnitus learn to live with it. Listening to soft background music helps some people to sleep better at night.

Teeth

Mary Anderson, DDS, draws a verbal picture in her article, "Portrait of Aging Teeth." As we grow older our teeth tend to darken. Actually, it's the dentin that darkens, a material underneath the tooth enamel. Drinking large quantities of coffee and smoking can make our teeth even darker.

The enamel on our teeth wears down after years of chewing. Our salivary glands may produce less saliva. "Saliva is very important to the fight against dental decay—it rinses the mouth, removing particles of food and decay-causing acids," writes Anderson. Aging people are more at risk for gum disease and tooth loss.

Kenneth Shay, DDS, MS, and Jonathan Ship, DMD, examine oral health in their study, "The Importance of Oral Health in the Older Patient." Their study has two purposes:

1. To alert other health professionals (non-dental) to oral disease in older people

2. To recruit other health professionals in disease prevention

The researchers attribute tooth loss to disease, not aging, and explain that "age alone does not seem to play a strong role in the impairments."

These days aging people are more apt to have their natural teeth. However, they may also have plaque, cavities, gum disease, and something called "attachment loss." Dentists define this as the loss of connective tissue between the cementum part of the tooth and the bone. Our teeth also crack and break more easily.

It's important to have regular checkups and cleanings. While I am at the dentist's office I address a reminder postcard. The postcard tells me when it's time for my next checkup. Regular dental care is preventive medicine for the years ahead.

As we get older we have fewer taste buds and, therefore, a diminished sense of taste. Food may taste more bland to you. According to Dr. Claire Murphy of the San Diego University Medical Center, "Taste alerts the brain to the presence of sweet, sour, bitter, and salty substances." In her study, "Nutrition and Chemosensory Perception in the Elderly," Murphy says elderly people are less able to perceive bitterness. This is important because bitter herbs and spices are often used as flavor enhancers in mixes and made-from-scratch recipes.

You may find yourself craving salt and sugar more than when you were younger. Joseph Stevens and William Cain discuss something called "mixture suppression" in their study, "Changes in Taste and Flavor in Aging." When we eat, we respond to a mixture of tastes: saltiness, sourness, bitterness, specific ingredients, seasonings, and fat. "One component of a mixture of tastes can mask or mute other components," and the result is mixture suppression.

How does this affect our sense of taste? Elderly people may need twice as much salt as young people just to detect its presence in food. "Losses of both smell and taste can seriously disturb the flavor world of the aged person," the researchers note.

Environment also influences our appreciation of food. A friend of mine recently moved into a retirement community with assisted living benefits. One of these benefits is dinner. All of the food is made on the premises, including crusty breads, savory roasts, and fruit pies, yet my friend won't eat in the dining room. "They can give it [the food] any fancy name they want to, Peach Surprise, whatever," she declared. "It all tastes the same to me." My friend was really saying that she missed her own home and the kitchen she loved so much. I can understand her feelings.

Doctors have become more aware of the damaging effects of the sun. Simply put, the sun ages our skin. Bruce Beacham, MD, takes a look at skin problems in his study, "Common Dermatoses in the Elderly." Some common skin problems in aging people are decreased sensation, irregular pigmentation, skin pallor/laxity, and dermatitis.

Beacham explains that aging skin may feel rougher.

Long-term smokers have grayish-looking skin. In fact, doctors can tell by the pallor of the skin if their patients are smokers. Aging skin bruises more easily and the bruises take longer to heal. Two of the most obvious skin changes are wrinkles and rosacea.

Thirteen million people in the United States have rosacea, a chronic skin disorder that causes redness and dermatitis. Thomas Zuber of Michigan State University in East Lansing, Michigan, describes the disorder in his study, "Rosacea: Beyond the First Blush." The causes of rosacea are unknown, Zuber explains, although doctors know it strikes fair-skinned, middle-aged people.

Rosacea may look like adult acne. The difference is that it can lead to dry eyes, conjunctivitis, corneal problems, and bulbous noses. W.C. Fields, the famous star of silent films, was known for his rosacea nose. Having a big red nose isn't any fun, and it's embarrassing, as a 60-year-old grandmother discovered.

"My rosacea is getting worse by the week. Blotches here, veins there. I don't want to look like W.C. Fields," Esther complained. "Why, some people even think I'm an alcoholic." Esther is not a paranoid person.

Rosacea patients are often mistaken for alcoholics because of veins that appear on and near the nose.

According to Zuber, rosacea strikes more women then men. "Some experts believe it is primarily a vascular disorder because of the prominent blood vessels, erythema, and flushing." Treatment options include:

- Avoiding sun exposure
- Avoiding very hot water
- Avoiding facial scrubs/abrasives
- Watching consumption of hot liquids
- Antibiotics
- Topical lotions and creams

Diane Thiboutot, MD, author of a study called "Acne Rosacea," thinks patients with rosacea should also avoid spicy foods and alcohol. Laser treatment may be indicated for some skin lesions. Thiboutot also says women who have rosacea may want to wear makeup that has a slightly greenish tint.

Department stores don't carry this makeup, but your dermatologist should be able to write you a prescription for it. Concealing makeup and cover sticks may also be helpful. Use a gentle motion when you remove makeup from your face and dry your skin gently.

Bones

A line in a popular American spiritual talks about "them bones, them bones, them dry bones." Aging people may not have dry bones, but they may have thinning bones, or osteoporosis. This disease is caused by a lack of essential nutrients, hormone imbalance, and lack of exercise.

Common symptoms of the disease are cited in an Associated Press article by Lauran Neergaard, titled "FDA Panel Recommends Osteoporosis Drug." The symptoms include bone and back pain, height loss, cramping in legs and feet (especially at night), a humped back, extreme fatigue, and bone fractures.

Fortunately, osteoporosis is a preventable and treatable disease. Journalist Delia O'Hara details some of the medical advances in her article, "Osteoporosis," published in the *American Medical News*. Doctors now know that osteoporosis isn't an inevitable result of aging.

They also know that many people, especially teens, aren't getting the calcium they need to prevent osteoporosis later in life. "The World Health Organization defines low bone mass as mineral density measuring at least one standard deviation below the mean for normal 30-year-old women, and osteoporosis as bone mass measuring at least 2.5 standard deviations below the mean," writes O'Hara.

If this standard is applied to the American population some 8 to 10 million women have osteoporosis. Few of these cases are diagnosed. O'Hara says prevention is the key, "but the sheer size of the at risk population poses a major obstacle." An estimated 85 percent of the girls in our country don't get their daily calcium requirement.

How much calcium is enough? The National Institutes of Health recommends 1,000 milligrams of calcium per day for women ages 25 to 50 and 1,500 milligrams for women ages 50 to 65. Women who are 65 years old or older and on estrogen need 1,500 milligrams of calcium per day.

Education has to start early in childhood. We can make sure that we get enough calcium, our children get enough, and our grandchildren get enough. And we can take these prevention steps:

- Exercise (including weight-bearing exercise)
- Hormone replacement therapy
- Bone density tests
- Medication tracking (some prescription drugs can affect bone density)
- Physical therapy

Right now six states have laws on the books that mandate insurance companies to pay for bone density tests in at-risk patients. More people would probably be screened if they had insurance coverage. Osteoporosis isn't limited to women, men have it as well, and you may have seen elderly men who have hunched backs.

Heart

Heart disease continues to be the number one killer in our country. Many people don't even know they have heart disease, and the tragic death of Sergei Grinkov, the Russian ice skater, is proof of this. Nobody knew, least of all the skater himself, that he had a faulty heart valve.

As we get older we may have skipped heartbeats, fast beats, and arrhythmias. Arrhythmias have dozens of causes. Some are caused by heart defects and others are caused by medicine, a lesson I learned the hard way.

My husband and I had been invited out to dinner. Because I had been plagued by a cold all week, I took a popular cold remedy to stop my nose from running. To counter my sleepiness I drank two cups of coffee (half decaf, half regular) before dinner. I had wine with my meal and another cup of coffee afterwards.

Without any warning, I felt as if I might faint, and rolled sideways on the bench. My husband, father-in-law, and brother-in-law rushed to my side. From a distance I heard my father-in-law say, "I can't get a pulse." These were not the words I wanted to hear.

My husband pressed an artery in my neck that restored my heartbeat to normal. Fifteen minutes later I was able to sit up and walk to the car with assistance. When I got home I read the fine print on the medicine box. Sure enough, there was a warning about taking the medicine with coffee and/or alcohol.

I will never make this mistake again. Thank goodness I knew my heart was fine because I had undergone a battery of tests a few weeks before. The technician had let me watch the progress of the test on the monitor screen. Seeing the steady pumping action of my heart had been reassuring.

Coronary heart disease is the most prevalent disease in aging people. Arteries gradually become clogged with fatty deposits (cholesterol). Smoking also makes the arteries narrower. These arterial changes force the heart to work harder and the blood pressure goes up.

The best thing we can do to prevent heart disease is to take care of ourselves. We can have regular physical exams, eat a healthy diet, and exercise regularly. Doctors recommend a minimum of 30 minutes four times a week. This includes five minutes of warm-up time and five minutes of cool-down time.

Lungs

Our lungs change as we get older. As Mark Beers, MD, and Stephen Urice, PhD, JD, note in their book, *Aging In Good Health,* there is less air movement with each breath as we get older. Less oxygen is routed through the blood system. Strenuous exercise gets more difficult as we age, and we may have breathing problems at high altitudes.

Chronic Obstructive Pulmonary Disease, commonly called emphysema, also makes breathing more difficult. It starts with "smokers cough" (bronchitis) and develops into obstructive pulmonary disease. The lung's ability to move air diminishes gradually and breathing becomes labored.

Physically inactive people also may have breathing problems. Experts recommend a program of regular aerobic exercise. The word aerobic is important because it implies that your heart rate reaches a certain number of beats per minute for a certain amount of time. Your aerobic rate is determined by age.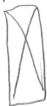

Kidneys

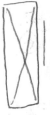

Beers and Urice go on to say that our kidneys shrink with age. There is decreased blood flow to the kidneys and our urine may be more concentrated, especially if we don't drink enough water. Many of us drink too many caffeinated beverages, which are diuretics, and eliminate water from our bodies.

Our ability to eliminate salt may also decrease. A physical exam may reveal an abnormal salt level in the body. Dietitians say our tolerance to salt is a conditioned response; the more we eat, the more we want. Chapter Four, "We Can Age Successfully," offers tips for cutting salt in your diet.

Veins

Varicose veins may develop early in life and both men and women have them. According to a Mayo Clinic Health Letter article, "Varicose Veins," the condition may be an inherited trait. "About 15 percent of American adults eventually develop them," the article notes. Weakened vein walls and valves are the two main causes of varicose veins.

The symptoms may be familiar to you: aching legs, bulging veins, dry/itchy skin, vein inflammation, and open sores (ulcers). Varicose veins can get worse during pregnancy. Some self-help tips, according to the Mayo Clinic Health Letter, are:

- Wearing support stockings
- Walking
- Raising your legs
- Getting up and moving around
- Avoiding tight girdles/panty girdles (I would add tight socks to this list.)
- Controlling weight

Putting lotion on varicose veins has also helped many

people. Lotion prevents the dry skin from ulcerating over the varicose veins. The idea is to keep the skin as healthy as possible. Apply lotion in the morning and at night if you live in a cold climate.

Digestion

Chili that tasted good when you were in your 20s may cause indigestion when you're in your 40s. Another problem, at least in my community, is that restaurants serve huge portions—18-ounce steaks, mountains of French fries, salads that would feed a small family. Visitors, especially those from Europe, are shocked at the portion sizes. I guess there's a reason why television ads promise heartburn relief.

Eating smaller portions helps to prevent indigestion. Order a large steak and share it. A friend of mine eats half her dinner and takes the rest home for the next day. Avoid eating large meals at night. There are good antacids on the market, but make sure you follow the product directions.

Instead of ordering spicy food, you may want to order something bland, such as broiled fish. Eat slowly and chew each mouthful of food several times. Steer clear of gas-producing foods, such as lima beans, baked beans, and hummus. You may also want to avoid soybeans.

An inexpensive filler and stabilizer, soybeans are often a hidden ingredient in foods. You may be surprised at the foods that contain soy: ice cream, frozen pizza, canned soups, and baked goods. Soybeans are listed on product labels as soy flour, soy protein, soy protein isolate, hydrolized vegetable protein, textured vegetable protein (TVP), and vegetable protein meal.

To avoid a gassy stomach you might want to take Beano before meals. The enzyme supplement is available in tablet and liquid form. Nonprescription gas tablets may also help you.

Dizziness and Spells

This heading may remind you of dramas in which the heroine faints gracefully onto a flowered couch. Actually, dizzy spells are a common complaint in aging people. Philip Sloane, MD, MPH, writes about these problems in his study, "Evaluation and Management of Dizziness in the Older Patient."

Sloane explains that almost all cases of dizziness in aging people are due to disease, and not to "normal aging." Many diseases cause dizziness, among them anemia, physical deconditioning, strokes, and low blood pressure. According to "Spells," an article published in the *Mayo Clinic Health Letter*, dizziness and spells are different.

Spell is a catch-all term used by medical professionals to "describe a variety of physical symptoms that occur for no apparent reason." The article explains that spells have three common factors:

1. They come on suddenly.

2. They last for an indefinite period of time.

3. They are usually months apart.

Spells may be caused by cardiovascular, psychological, neurological, or hormonal problems, or they may be related to drugs, food intolerance, or allergy. There are other causes of dizziness and one of them is Benign Positional Vertigo, or BVP.

Some aging people literally have rocks in their heads. Calcium crystals in the inner ear, which are like little rocks, work their way into the wrong ear channels. The results are dizziness, loss of balance, and in some cases, nausea. Doctors treat this condition with a Canalith Repositioning Maneuver. With this maneuver the patient is rotated to shake the calcium deposits loose. You have to wear a neck collar overnight and sleep upright to help the calcium deposits to stabilize. If you lie down accidentally (a frequent problem)

the maneuver must be repeated. The maneuver may also
have to be repeated if other calcium deposits shake loose.

Report any spells or bouts of dizziness to your doctor.

Before doctors can identify the cause of your dizziness
you may have to go through a battery of tests. Even then,
doctors may not be sure of the cause, and will continue to
monitor your health. Menopause causes dizzy spells for
some people.

Menopause

Women may consider menopause the demarcation line between youth and old age. The first hot flash signals the
change and from then on, we may think of ourselves as old.
Just because your mother went through menopause in her
mid-50s doesn't mean you will experience it at the same
time. The average age for the onset of menopause is 48.

Symptoms of menopause include the infamous hot
flashes, irritability, sleep problems, bloating, dry eyes, and
vaginal dryness. The hot flashes can be so severe that they
cause fainting. Enter the era of hormone replacement therapy. You may know about HRT but you may not know that
the dosage has to be adjusted to your health needs. An article in the *Mayo Clinic Women's HealthSource,* "Hormone
Replacement Therapy," tells women to work with their
health care providers to customize their therapy.

There are distinct advantages to HRT; it protects against
uterine cancer and bone degeneration, and some doctors
think it sparks creative brain activity. Chapter Five, "Sexuality, Intimacy, and Love" contains more information on
menopause.

Boston Globe columnist Ellen Goodman writes about
menopause in her column, "Meno—the Pause That Refreshes." She says aging women were often dismissed in the
past because they were considered obsolete. Times are
changing. Goodman cites a recent anthropological study of

hunter-gatherers in Tanzania that portrays older women as the breadwinners.

Goodman thinks nature planned for women to be older and wiser. "When childbearing ends, gear up to the job of making life better for the whole clan," she writes. There is plenty to do even if we don't work outside the home. See Chapter Six, "Making a Difference," for more information on using time wisely.

Prostate Disease

If they live long enough most men get prostate disease. The prostate gland tends to enlarge with age, according to an article in the *Mayo Clinic Health Letter.* "More than half of men older than age 50, and 80 percent of men in their 70s, experience prostate enlargement," the article notes.

Men with prostate disease may not be able to empty their bladders fully, urinate more often, find it hard to postpone urination, have weak urinary output, strain to urinate, and get up several times at night to void. Urine buildup can lead to bladder infections.

Treatment options include drug therapy with alpha blockers, which relax muscle tissue, and hormone suppressers, which suppress testosterone. Another article in the *Mayo Clinic Health Letter* reports "surgery is still the mainstay of treatment." This surgery, called transurethral resection of the prostate, is performed by a urologist.

Incontinence

Incontinence is a common problem in aging people. Losing bladder and/or bowel control is embarrassing and worrisome. Stress incontinence—loss of control due to coughing, laughing, or exertion—is particularly embarrassing. The causes of incontinence include weak muscles, bladder infections, uncontrolled diabetes, prostate disease, diarrhea, and medication.

As we grow older, we may not be able to delay elimination as we did when we were younger. Digestive problems may also cause incontinence. Contact your doctor if you have any problems with leaking or soiling. All symptoms should be checked out carefully. "Incontinence," an article published in the *Mayo Clinic Health Letter,* says a variety of treatments are available:

- Behavior modification
- Pelvic floor exercises (commonly called Kegels)
- Medications
- Bulking agents (substances injected into the lining of the urethra)
- Urethral plug for women
- Urethral patch for women
- Pessary (device that is put into the vagina)
- Surgery

There are a growing number of treatments for incontinence, the article says, including a device implanted in the spine. Absorbent pads and underwear are also available. Doctors and medical manufacturers continue to look for solutions to incontinence.

Stamina

Stamina varies from person to person like the other physical aspects of aging. One thing is sure, lack of exercise is a major health problem in America. We park the car close to the mall entrance so we don't have to walk. We use the remote control to change the channels on the TV. The more sedentary we become, the more out of condition we become.

Muscle loss contributes to deconditioning. After age 65 men lose about 10 percent of their muscle capacity, according to the Mayo Clinic, women a little less. Exercise is one solution to the problem.

Instead of choosing the easiest route, let's choose the exercise route. Park at the back of the lot and walk to the mall entrance. Turn off the TV for the weekend and get outdoors. Take the stairs instead of the elevator. Better yet, we can exercise with our grandchildren.

The people who responded to my survey had lots to say about the physical aspects of aging. Aches and pains were the symptoms listed most often. Other symptoms include:

- creaky knees and swollen joints
- arthritis
- skin problems
- osteoporosis
- breakdown of body parts
- failing eyesight/hearing
- loss of stamina

On her survey form a friend of mine wrote, "My body from head on down is going south." Many of us have made the same observation. From face, to chest, to tummy, to thighs, our bodies are shifting downward. It seems no body part is immune from the trend and we are amazed at the changes we see.

"Going South"

Our faces may start to resemble the faces we have seen in family photo albums. Lips wrinkle. Cheeks sag. Hairlines recede. The same friend who said her body was going south said her face was going in the same direction. This causes some people to misjudge her.

"My features are sagging and people think I'm angry," she explained. "I'm not angry, it's my sagging facial muscles. What can I do? I'm not going to have plastic surgery, and forcing myself to smile all day is tiring."

We don't have to smile all day, but we have things to smile about. Researchers are learning more about the aging process. Some speculate that lifestyle, diet, and environment account for 65 percent of longevity, and genetics for only 35 percent. I think these are startling statistics. If nothing else, the statistics may force us to take stock of our lifestyles.

"What we do in our 20s, 30s, and 40s can have a huge impact on how fast we age," writes Maureen West of the *New York Times* News Service. In her article, "Lifetime of Habits Determine Differences in the Aging Process," West says we can live long, healthy lives "if care has been taken earlier." So take care of yourself and follow these smart aging tips.

Smart Aging Tips

- Focus on the physical positives in your life.
- Monitor weight gain and be aware of how many calories you consume each day.
- Have your vision checked and wear sunglasses.
- Have your hearing checked and carry earplugs with you.
- Visit the dentist regularly.
- Have your doctor check any skin changes you see.
- Wear sunscreen and a protective hat when you are outdoors.
- Get a bone density test if you are female.
- Eat enough calcium.
- Give up smoking.
- Drink enough water.
- Exercise regularly.
- Report dizziness and other spells to your physician.
- Customize hormone replacement therapy to your body's responses and needs.

3

Medical Tests That Could Save Your Life

The idea of medical tests upsets some people, especially if they don't know what the tests involve. But every day, in our country and around the world, medical tests are saving lives. It is hard to keep up with the advances in medicine because they are coming so fast.

There are hundreds, if not thousands, of medical tests. This chapter would be a book if I listed all of them, so I have focused on these topics:

- High-tech tests
- Better test analysis
- Imaging (Ultrasound, Magnetic Resonance Imaging, Computerized Tomography, Radionuclide Scanning)
- Old tests, new importance
- Mammograms
- Genetics and gene therapy
- Checkups

This chapter is written from a preventive medicine standpoint. Doctors hope we will get the tests we need. All too often, however, we let our tests lapse. Many of us, especially women, are not even getting basic medical tests, such as blood pressure. These people may be putting their lives at risk.

High-Tech Tests

One day, when I was in a hospital coffee shop, I heard a woman say, "I'm not taking that test." She poured cream into her coffee, stirred it nervously, and added, "I don't want to hear the results." While I can understand this woman's fear, I find it difficult to understand her self-neglect.

Whatever the test was, it could be the difference between life and death; consider a pap smear or mammogram, for example. Cox News Service journalist Amanda Husted writes about these tests in her article, "Many Women Avoid Two Tests That Could Save Their Lives." She lists the excuses women give for avoiding the tests:

- Loss of time (at home and work)
- Think the test isn't important
- Cost of the test
- Afraid to hear results (like the woman in the coffee shop)

Lack of child care may prevent some women from getting the medical tests. Fear of the unknown may be another reason. Odd-looking machines with monitor screens, flashing lights, and loud buzzers can scare anyone. Still, the avoidance statistics on women are worrisome.

Thirty-seven percent of American women failed to get a pap smear in 1996, Husted reports, and roughly one out of five women over 50 failed to get a mammogram. Yet Husted says the tests "take about the same amount of time as a hair cut." Pap smears and mammograms are uncomfortable, but I have them anyway.

Once you are familiar with a test you may be less fearful of it. You'll know how to prepare for the test and what to expect.

Although blood pressure testing is not new, it continues to be a trend in medicine. The blood pressure test is a staple of medicine, one of the first tests in a routine physical exam. Usually blood pressure tests are done in a doctor's office.

Better Test Analysis

In the past doctors measured blood pressure with a blood pressure cuff. Now they often use electronic machines. Worrying about a blood pressure test can actually raise your blood pressure. Doctors call this response "white coat hypertension."

Associated Press writer Brenda Coleman discusses the response in her article, "Monitor Spots 'White-Coat' Hypertension." About 20 percent of the patients who have their blood pressure taken in a doctor's office have higher readings. "Just being in a doctor's office is enough to send millions of people's blood pressure soaring," she writes.

Belgian researchers are working on a machine that can tell the difference between white coat hypertension and actual high blood pressure. Designed to be used in non-medical settings, the machine is about the size of a portable radio. Researchers know the cost of the machine may inhibit sales and are trying to reduce this cost.

Thomas Pickering, MD, writes about white-coat hypertension in an editorial titled, "A New Role for Ambulatory Blood Pressure Monitoring?" Experts think blood pressure should be measured in two places, according to Pickering, at home and in a medical setting.

"There is also evidence that if patients with white-coat hypertension are started on medication, the office BP is reduced but not the BP during the rest of the day."

Inexpensive home blood pressure monitors are now available. The monitor gives you a means of tracking the fluctuations in your blood pressure. Some monitors store and print out data. Having a home blood pressure monitor is not only reassuring, it may save you a visit to the doctor's office.

Imaging

Imaging techniques, such as ultrasound, magnetic resonance imaging, computerized tomography (CT scan), and radionuclide scanning are the new staples of medicine. Doctors use these tests to obtain detailed, graphic information about the body. Imaging techniques are getting better all the time.

ULTRASOUND

The ultrasound test has many advantages and they are listed in an article called, "Diagnostic Ultrasound," published in the *Mayo Clinic Health Letter*. First, and perhaps foremost in your mind, ultrasound is a noninvasive test. No needles, no surgery, no radiation. The test is versatile and has no side effects.

Three types of ultrasound are available: gray-scale, Doppler, and duplex Doppler. Gray-scale ultrasound is used to show internal organs. Doppler ultrasound is used to analyze blood flow. Duplex Doppler combines gray-scale and Doppler to picture anatomy and blood flow. Magnetic resonance imaging (MRI) is another non-invasive imaging test.

MAGNETIC RESONANCE IMAGING

The test involves magnetizing the body and sending a radio signal to orient the body's hydrogen atoms. Another radio signal is sent and the exiting signal reveals the structure of the body. MRI used to sound like Star Wars stuff to me, and while I appreciated its technical magic, I was afraid to take the test.

Every time I thought about the test I had a mental image of a coffin. Would I be able to lie in an enclosed cylinder for

40 minutes? Would I be able to lie perfectly still? Would I make a fool of myself? "I'm afraid I'll get claustrophobic," I told my doctor.

A brilliant, cheerful, and compassionate woman, she gave me a prescription for three valium. I was instructed to take one pill the day before the MRI to see how I tolerated the medicine. The second pill was to be taken just before the test and the third only if necessary.

"It's a good idea to get there early," she said.

The day before the test, however, I was so busy with other tests that I didn't have time to take the trial pill. I took the pill just before I arrived at the MRI appointment desk. Other patients were waiting and the tests seemed to be progressing slowly.

Afraid that my valium would wear off before the test, I approached the desk. "I h-a-v-e t-aaaa-k-e-n a p-r-e-s-c-r-iiiii-b-e-d v-aaaa-l-i-u-m," I said. "It m-aaa-y be w-e-a-r-i-n-ggggg offffff. Do you think I s-h-oooo-u-l-d t-a-k-e a-n-o-t-h-e-rrrr?" For some reason the secretaries were staring at me with their mouths open.

"No!" they exclaimed in unison. "We'll get you in soon."

Needless to say, I had no trouble with the test. It seems the stories I had heard were exaggerated. The MRI chamber was large, well lit, and equipped with a mirror, and the technician stayed in contact with me via intercom. During my MRI I mentally revised this book to keep my mind off the test. You could do something similar.

MRI machines continue to improve. Open-sided machines are available for plus-size people and those who have claustrophobia. Doctors don't think the resolution is as good, however. You may have to do work your way through the yellow pages to find a facility that has open-sided machines.

I was glad I had the MRI, and the results were encouraging. This story illustrates the importance of keeping an open mind. If you have any questions about the test, ask the doctors or the medical technician. Even if you think your questions sound silly, ask them, because all of your questions are valid.

COMPUTERIZED TOMOGRAPHY

Another imaging test is computerized tomography (CT), or cat scan, as medical professionals call it. According to the editors of the 1998 *Current Medical Diagnosis & Treatment,* computerized tomography images the heart and, with the use of a contrast medium, the vascular system. Its main application is with pericardial disease.

There are two kinds of CT scans: x-ray and electron beam. Immatron uses an electron beam to "spiral" through the body and these spirals are photographed. Doctors can do things with a CT scan that they cannot do with magnetic resonance imaging, such as using iodine as a contrast agent.

RADIONUCLIDE SCANNING

Radionuclide scanning is yet another form of imaging. It involves the use of nuclear isotopes to diagnose and treat disease. This type of imaging helps to diagnose prostate cancer, cardiomyopathy, heart disease, pulmonary hypertension, pulmonary embolism (blood clots), myocardial infarction, and renal disease.

Doctors may find clues to disease with radionuclide scanning that other tests missed. For example, prostate cancer is often revealed by back pain. According to the 1998 *Current Medical Diagnosis & Treatment,* "Radionuclide bone scan is conventional to plain skeletal x-rays in detecting bony metasteses. Most prostatic cancer metasteses are multiple and are most commonly localized in the axial skeleton."

Of course, diagnosis doesn't hinge upon one test. Doctors will use a variety of tests to make a diagnosis.

Nuclear medicine continues to be a growing trend in

medicine. Some tests aren't new, such as the colon test, yet they have new importance in the diagnosis of disease.

Old Tests, New Importance

The top three killers in the United States are heart disease, stroke, and cancer, including colon cancer. A colon test is one of the most important tests you can have after age 50 and doctors are relying on it more than ever. NBC news medical correspondent and writer, Nancy Snyderman, MD, writes about this test in her article, "Colon Cancer: Stopping a Killer in Our Midst."

COLON TEST

Snyderman tells about her family's history of colon cancer. This history prompted Snyderman's father, a surgeon, to get yearly colon exams. "The testing paid off," she writes. "My father's cancer was detected early, the tumor was removed immediately, and he was cured."

Snyderman worries about her own risk of colon cancer. Colon polyps have been discovered and surgically removed. Although the polyps were noncancerous, she says they warn her that she "can't let my guard down."

You have to fast and clean your body with enemas and laxatives before the test. Follow the pretest guidelines carefully. Some patients (including me) have had an adverse reaction to the enema-laxative series. Tell your doctor if this happens to you.

Uncomfortable as it is, I know the colon test is a health necessity. As I was entering the dressing room, the woman next to me was leaving. "I have this test every year," she confided. "Every year they find polyps and I have surgery. This test keeps saving my life."

More lives could be saved if people had regular colon tests. The test takes about 30 minutes and you may be able to watch its progress on a monitor screen. After age 50 the risk factor for colon cancer doubles. There are other risk factors, according to "Colon Cancer Screening," published in the *Mayo Clinic Health Letter,* such as:

- Close relative(s) who have colon polyps
- Inflammatory bowel disease
- High-fat, low-fiber diet
- Medical history of colon polyps

In some instances the doctor recommends a colonoscopy. This surgical procedure is performed under moderate anesthesia. A flexible endoscope is inserted into the colon. The endoscope shows the colon's interior lining and allows your doctor to check for polyps. Early detection of polyps is a weapon against colon cancer.

Exercise is another weapon, according to Associated Press writer Ira Dreyfuss. The title of her article, "Women Reduce Their Risk of Colon Cancer Through Exercise," states the premise clearly. Dreyfuss explains, "Walking at a normal or brisk pace for an hour per day is associated with a 46 percent reduction in risk of the No. 3 cancer killer of women in the United States."

Your risk goes down even if you only walk for a half hour. Dreyfuss says doctors don't know why exercise reduces the risk of colon cancer, but think it may speed waste materials through the bowel. Walking is still the best form of exercise.

ULCER TEST

Doctors used to think ulcers were caused by stress alone. Now they think ulcers may be caused by *H. Pylori* bacteria. For years doctors have relied on endoscopy to detect ulcers, an invasive procedure that involves swallowing a tube.

Mayo Medical Laboratories has come up with a noninvasive, less expensive test. Luke Shockman describes the test in his *Rochester Post-Bulletin* article, "Ulcers an Easy Target." The 30-minute test involves eating pudding to coat the lining of the stomach, drinking a solution, and then exhaling into a container. Doctors can tell, by analyzing your breath, if you have ulcers. The Food and Drug Administration has approved the test.

Mayo Clinic researchers think the test will cut down on the number of patients who get antibiotics. The test will also cut your medical bills, according to Shockman. Endoscopy costs anywhere from $1,200 to $2,000, whereas the breath test costs about $360.

BONE DENSITY

Associated Press journalist Lauran Neergaard tells about the advances in bone testing in her article, "Test Helps Diagnose Thin Bones." Not only are the tests for osteoporosis getting easier and cheaper, Neergaard says they're getting better. The Food and Drug Administration has improved the Sahara Clinical Bone Sonometer test, which uses ultrasound instead of x-rays.

This test will help millions of women, Neergaard says, and they "can now simply slide a foot into a little machine and learn minutes later if their bones are dangerously thin." The Sahara test is portable, small (about the size of a laser printer) and painless.

MAMMOGRAM

Although it has been around for years, breast cancer screening has become even more important. Women who are 50 years old or older should have annual mammograms. Women between the ages of 40 and 49 should have a mammogram every two years. But some researchers have different opinions on when to have a mammogram.

"Mammograms: When to Start Screening," an article in the *Mayo Clinic Women's HealthSource,* says regular screening at age 40 makes good health sense. The article asks women to think about paying for a mammogram if their insurance plans don't cover them. A mammogram can detect a lump in the breast long before you can feel it.

Choose a medical facility that is certified by the U.S. Food and Drug Administration when you make an appointment. To find the facility nearest you, call the Cancer Information Service at 800-4-CANCER.

Breast self-examinations have also become a weapon against cancer. Are you confused about breast self-exams? A plastic shower card from the American Cancer Society tells you how to do it. Hang the card on the shower nozzle to remind yourself about the exam. Call 800-ACS-2345 to get your free card.

GLAUCOMA TEST

Although a glaucoma test may not save your life, it may save your sight. Glaucoma changes the eye's lens, hardening what is called the globe of the eye. The disease restricts vision, and patients who have it may see halos around light bulbs and other artificial lighting. If glaucoma isn't treated the patient may go blind.

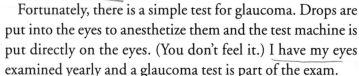

Fortunately, there is a simple test for glaucoma. Drops are put into the eyes to anesthetize them and the test machine is put directly on the eyes. (You don't feel it.) I have my eyes examined yearly and a glaucoma test is part of the exam.

Genetics

The most amazing medical breakthrough of the century may be genetic engineering. Researchers have learned how to clone animals and how to improve crops, and they are always working on ways to combat major diseases. Jeff Lyon writes about genetics and gene therapy in his article, "Amazing Medical Breakthroughs."

Lyon says gene therapy is "a catchall term for a crunch of elegant methodologies that are in the works to diagnose, prevent and combat afflictions of almost every kind." He thinks of gene therapy as a kind of medical transplant and tells how some of the therapies may be used.

Healthy genes may be given to someone who has faulty genes. According to Lyon, most of the current trials are for cancer, and treatments may be available for general use within the next few years.

Genes may be used for immunotherapy, that is, to prevent someone from getting a disease. Lastly, gene therapy may be used for pharmacological treatment. More uses for gene therapy will be discovered as scientists uncover our genetic secrets. In a sense, researchers are "re-inventing" DNA. "Gene therapy is a startling new medical landscape that lies just beyond the millennium," writes Lyon.

Get a Checkup

It's been around for years, but an old-fashioned physical exam, or checkup, is one of the best ways to save your life. A checkup helps your doctor to prevent disease (measles, flu, etc.), identify disease early, and limit its harm. Doctors recommend four exams per decade when you are in your 40s, five exams per decade when you are in your 50s, and yearly exams after age 60. Apply this rule of thumb only if you are in good health. If you have a chronic illness, such as diabetes, you may have to see your doctor more often.

Anthony Galanos, MD, and his colleagues focus on checkups in their study, "The Comprehensive Assessment of Community Dwelling Elderly: Why Functional Status Is Not Enough." They urge health professionals to gather patient information from various sources: medical, cognitive, psychiatric, and functional. "It is not a matter of which is more important," they explain, "but rather of what useful information each contributes to an individual case."

Time passes more quickly as we get older. You may think you just had a checkup, only to discover it was years ago. That happened to me. So it's a good idea to write your appointment on the calendar and, if there is room, the tests you had. Making a follow-up appointment is also a good idea. When you are in the doctor's office ask about your immunizations. You may need a tetanus booster, flu shot, or pneumonia vaccination. Staying up to date on your immunizations helps you to stay in good health.

Quackery

Finally, as you do your best to stay healthy, know that medical quackery has become blatant. People who haven't been to an accredited college or university are practicing medicine and physical therapy. They share a common goal and that is profit.

Fitness experts permeate the television airwaves. One woman wears a clip-on microphone and keeps telling viewers to "breathe out." Of course we're going to breathe out. Does she think we are going to hold our breath until we faint?

Liz Neporent reviews some of the exercise shows in her article, "Living-Room Leg Lifts: A Guide to TV Exercise Shows." While she gives some shows top ratings, Neporent blasts others for their content. The stars of one show are out of step with one another, she comments, and another show is rated as "beefcake and enough silicone to qualify as 'Baywatch' extras."

Self-proclaimed diet experts are hawking their plans on television. Some of these people have no nutritional training at all. You may drop pounds on their diets, but body chemistry is complex, and you may also drop dead. Talk with your doctor before you go on a diet or take any diet pills.

Only qualified physicians are allowed to write prescriptions. Other health professionals, who are not medical doctors, are asking for these privileges. I don't know about you, but I want the person who writes my prescriptions to have had years of chemistry, not a quick crash course.

If you have any concerns about the health professional you are seeing, contact your local medical and/or dental society. Or call the American Dental Association at 1-800-621-8099 or the American Medical Association at 1-800-458-5736. Both associations are based in Chicago.

Preventive Services Tests

If there is a moral to this chapter, it is to get the tests you need. These tests depend on your family history, medical history, your lifestyle, where you live, and your doctor's assessment. While doctors have different opinions on test timing, they agree on the benefits of preventive tests.

What tests do you need and when do you need them? You will find some general guidelines at the end of the chapter. Talk with your doctor about the medical tests he or she recommends. HMOs and government plans, such as Medicare, have varying test standards. Your tests may, or may not, be covered by your insurance plan.

Medical tests and advances can help us to live longer, healthier lives. We must keep up with the breakthroughs if we are to benefit from them, so watch for newspaper and magazine articles. Check the Internet for more information. Friends may also have helpful information to share with you.

Smart Aging Tips

- Try to get the medical tests you need.
- Buy a home monitor if you have high blood pressure.
- Talk to your doctor if you have white-coat hypertension.
- Face your medical fears and discuss them with health professionals.
- Have a colon test.
- Be aware of test improvements.
- Be on the lookout for quackery.
- Have regular checkups as recommended by your doctor.
- Keep your tests current.
- Call national medical agencies for more information. (See list in the appendix.)

What Tests, What Age?

Test	Age 35–49	Age 50–65	Age 66+
Blood pressure check	Every 1–2 years if normal	Same	Yearly
Chest x-ray	Every 1–2 years if normal	Same	Yearly
Total cholesterol, HDL ("good cholesterol") and Triglycerides	Every 5 yrs. if normal	Same	Yearly
Pap smear*	Yearly, if normal, for 3 years. Then every 3 years.	Yearly if any abnormal cells are detected.	Consult your doctor.
Mammogram	Every 1–2 years age 40–49; yearly if you have a family history of breast cancer	Yearly	Consult your doctor
Bone density test	Per doctor's orders	Every 2 yrs.	Consult your doctor

*The Mayo Clinic recommends yearly pap smears if you have had more than two sexual partners in your lifetime, you were under age 18 when you had intercourse for the first time, have a history of sexually transmitted diseases, or if you are a smoker. If your partner has a sexually transmitted disease you need yearly pap smears.

What Tests, What Age? (continued)

Test	Age 35–49	Age 50–65	Age 66+
Glaucoma test	Per doctor's orders	Yearly	Yearly
Prostate check	Every visit to your doctor	Yearly	Yearly
Skin cancer check	Every visit to your doctor	Yearly if you live in a southern climate; every 6 months if you have had previous cancer	Same
Flexible sigmoidoscopy	Every 5 yrs. if you have no polyps; if polyps develop every 3 yrs. or as directed by your doctor	Same	Consult your doctor
Colonoscopy	Every 3 yrs. if polyps develop or you have a strong family history of cancer	Same	Same
Fecal occult blood test	Per doctor's orders	Yearly	Yearly

Sources: Mayo Clinic, "Checkups: A Time for Action," *Mayo Clinic Women's HealthSource*, August 1997, p 6; *Mayo Clinic Preventive Services Clinic* (brochure); and U.S. government guidelines.

Smart Aging

4

We Can Age Successfully

"Successful aging" turns up in the medical literature time and again, and that is the origin of this chapter. Although the rate of aging varies from person to person, all of us may take steps to age successfully. Renee Solomon, DSW, and Monte Peterson, MD, detail these steps in their study, "Successful Aging: How to Help Your Patients Cope With Change."

Today's retirees have a third of their lives ahead of them, the researchers point out, "and they naturally want to live their remaining years as best they can." Eating right is an important step on the path to successful aging.

Eat Right

Good nutrition isn't a fad, it is a lifelong commitment. Joyce Keithley uses the phrase "eating right for life" in her study titled, "Promoting Good Nutrition: Using the Food Guide Pyramid in Clinical Practice." She cites some eye-opening statistics on obesity in our country.

One out of every four whites is obese. One out of every three blacks is obese. One out of every three Hispanics is obese. Even more worrisome is the fact that obese people are often malnourished. "It is not surprising, therefore, that as many as 50% of all patients admitted to hospitals are moderately or severely malnourished," Keithley reports.

What is eating right? Maciej Buchowski, PhD, and Ming Sun, PhD, set some dietary guidelines in their study, "Nutrition in Minority Elders: Current Problems and Future Directions." They recommend a diet with a fat content less than 30 percent, more vitamin B6, riboflavin, and vitamin D (found in fruits and vegetables), and rich in calcium.

As sensible as these guidelines sound, they may not get translated into action. Minority elders, including African Americans from the south who "have a strong sense of autonomy," may know what they should be eating but they don't eat it, according to the authors. They suggest replacing existing dietary fats with olive or canola oil.

When the food pyramid guidelines were first issued I didn't pay attention to them because I thought I was eating right. I was wrong. It turns out I wasn't getting enough fruits and vegetables. After I made this discovery I paid more attention to the guidelines.

The Food Pyramid

Can the food pyramid guidelines be applied to your life? Lori Wirth, BA, MHSE, tells how to use the pyramid in her study, "Plotting on the Food Pyramid: an Evaluation of Dietary Patterns." She describes a nutrition project at Oak Park High School in Gainesville, Florida. The project had three main parts.

First, students kept a detailed food diary that included brand names and serving sizes. Next, the students created personal food pyramids based on their diaries. Last, they evaluated their eating patterns in relation to the food pyramid.

Bread, rice, cereal, and pasta form the base of the pyramid. Fruits and vegetables (separated into two groups) form the next level. The next level is milk products, meat, poultry, fish, beans, and eggs. Fats, oils, and sweets form the tip of the pyramid. Students learned that some foods, such as cheese, fit into both the dairy and fat groups.

According to the U.S. Department of Agriculture, we need to eat 6 to 11 servings of bread, rice, cereal, and pasta per day. We need to eat 3 to 5 servings of fruits and vegetables. And we need to eat 2 to 3 servings of dairy foods and meat, including poultry, fish, and dried beans. Fats and oils should be used sparingly.

Some people are following the Mediterranean food pyramid, based on the eating patterns of Crete, Greece, and Southern Italy. Walter Willett and his colleagues spotlight the diet in their study, "Mediterranean Diet Pyramid: A Cultural Model for Healthy Eating." This diet uses fresh produce, grains, small amounts of fish and poultry, limited dairy products, and few or no eggs per week.

Unlike Northern European diets, which rely on animal fats for cooking, the Mediterranean diet relies on olive oil. Willett thinks olive oil has been shown to increase the high-density lipoproteins ("good cholesterol"), has stood the test of time, and brings out the flavor of fresh vegetables and legumes.

I love this diet. Offer me sweet onions, juicy tomatoes, crunchy peppers, fragrant fruit, crusty bread, and fresh garlic, and I'll follow you anywhere. Well, almost anywhere. Since I don't like strong olive oil, I use the extra light variety. Following the food pyramid is good preventive medicine.

In fact, preventing chronic disease was one of the original purposes of the pyramid. Unfortunately, meat and dairy producers lobbied against the pyramid and publication was halted in 1991. Marion Nestle, who is with the Department of Nutrition, Food, and Hotel Management at New York University, reviews the controversy in her article, "Food Lobbies, the Food Pyramid, and US Nutrition Policy." She thinks the controversy focuses new attention on an old problem—governmental protection of the public versus the rights of private business. Nestle also thinks the playing field is far from level. "What is at stake here is no less than the health of the public," she comments.

Following the food pyramid guidelines is a personal choice. I find the guidelines helpful and try to follow them each day. The guidelines help me to get the vitamins I need. Researchers continue to study the effects of vitamins on the body.

Vitamins

Researcher Jeffrey Blumberg, author of "The Requirement for Vitamins in Aging and Age-Associated Degenerative Conditions," writes, "The evidence is now undisputed that diet and nutrition are directly linked to many of the chronic diseases afflicting older adults and the elderly."

A study in the *Journal of the American Medical Association* (*JAMA*) by Eric Rimm, ScD, and his colleagues reports that folate and vitamin B_6 may help to prevent chronic heart disease. The study, "Folate and Vitamin B_6 from Diet and Supplements in Relation to Risk of Coronary Heart Disease Among Women," is based on questionnaires from 80,082 nurses.

The 1980 questionnaire covers a wide range of topics, including cold cereal, vitamin supplements (if used), number of vitamins taken per week, and portion sizes. For 14 years the researchers followed the study participants. "Risk of CHD [chronic heart disease] was lowest among women with the highest intake of both folate and vitamin B_6." Women who consumed alcohol in moderation benefited most from a high-folate diet.

New York Times News Service columnist Jane Brody comments on the study in her article, "Study: Folate, B-6 May Be Heart Healthy." According to Brody, the study suggests that eating more produce, grains, and B vitamins may be as important as quitting smoking, lowering our cholesterol, or controlling high blood pressure in preventing chronic heart disease.

Eric Rimm (the study's primary author) is quoted as saying, "The exciting news is that a substantial reduction in risk can be achieved easily, without a dramatic change in diet." Rimm advises eating fortified cereals, orange juice, bananas, leafy greens, chicken, and fish.

According to an article in the *Mayo Clinic Women's HealthSource*, "The Vitamin Controversy," some people need to take vitamin supplements. Those people include the elderly, dieters, those who have digestive diseases, alcohol abusers, and vegetarians.

Many people consider vitamins as a kind of dietary insurance. Can you take too many vitamins? Doctors say yes, especially if you take them by the handful, a practice some call "bulking." The extra vitamins may not help you as much as you think. With some exceptions, the kidneys eliminate extra vitamins from your body.

To put it bluntly, when you take too many vitamins you are flushing money down the toilet. Your best source of vitamins is a balanced diet. Plus, your body gets the roughage it needs to keep your bowels regular. Some doctors recommend daily doses of vitamin E and C to improve health.

More research is needed on the vitamin requirements of aging people. Robert Russell and Paolo Suter make this point in their study, "Vitamin Requirements of Elderly People: An Update." Vitamin research is a dynamic and changing field, the authors say, and may lead to changes in health care.

As scientists learn more about the link between vitamins and health, the Recommended Daily Allowances (RDA) will probably change. "There are data to indicate that the 1989 RDAS are too low for the elderly population," note Russell and Suter. So it may be wise to stay attuned to vitamin research.

Organic Foods

You may think you need to eat organic foods in order to eat right. Organic foods account for about 1 percent of food sales in the nation, according to an Associated Press article, "Standards on Labeling Foods as Organic Released Today." Food industry experts think this percentage will rise.

Widespread confusion about the word "organic" prompted the Agriculture Department to issue guidelines for its use on December 15, 1997. Raw food must be 100 percent organic in order to qualify for the department's seal. Processed foods must be 95 percent organic. And partially organic foods must be labeled "made with certain organic ingredients."

You will find organic foods in grocery stores, farmers' markets, and health food stores. Be prepared to pay more for these products, for that is often the case.

The Calcium Quotient

Eating calcium is another way to age successfully. "Osteoporosis," an article in the *Mayo Clinic Women's Health-Source,* says the disease kills more women in America than breast cancer. And Robert Heaney, MD, looks at the calcium issue in his article, "Age Considerations in Nutrient Needs for Bone Health: Older Adults."

Aging people exercise less, eat less, and have reduced estrogen levels. The net result is less calcium in the bones. Milk is one of the best sources of calcium. As Heaney writes, "Milk is a food—an inexpensive food—a food that costs less per calorie than the calcium-poor and vitamin D-poor foods it would displace if it were to be incorporated into an elderly person's diet."

Kim Painter discusses the new national calcium guidelines in her *USA Today* article, "New Calcium Advice: Eat More." Painter thinks the guidelines boil down to drinking milk and eating veggies "because if you don't your bones will suffer." Older women who are taking estrogen need to get enough calcium. Together, estrogen, calcium, and vitamin D help to prevent bone degeneration. The article ends with calcium statistics from the American Dietetic Association. A cup of plain nonfat yogurt, for example, contains 450 milligrams of calcium.

Grocery stores are stocking more calcium-fortified products, such as milk, orange juice, bread, and rice, but you may have to search for them. Some doctors recommend calcium carbonate (Tums, Titralac, etc.) as an additional source of calcium. My gynecologist said two extra-strength tablets per day, combined with a balanced diet, will supply me with enough calcium. I buy calcium carbonate in bulk at a warehouse club.

Hold the Salt

Using less salt is another step on the road to successful aging. Americans love salty foods, but some of us are salt sensitive, according to Francis Haddy, MD, PhD, and his colleagues. Their study, "Role of Dietary Salt in Hypertension" examines the relationship between salt and hypertension, the most common chronic disease in America.

Most of us can eat as much salt as we like, provided our kidneys work efficiently. Salt sensitive people and those who have hypertension need to watch their intake. Hypertension is nothing to fool with and, if untreated, can lead to disability, stroke, heart failure, and kidney failure. "Subjects that are older and have higher pressures seem to benefit more from a reduction in sodium intake," the researchers explain.

After my husband's aorta dissected in 1996 I became a member of the "salt police." I discovered that salt turns up in surprising places, such as seasoned pepper! Many foods, such as fish and milk, contain natural salt. So virtually everything we eat, including breads, muffins, salad dressings, and sauces, is made from scratch.

We eat less than 2 grams of salt per day, something that is hard to do when we eat out. Reducing salt takes careful planning. A *Mayo Clinic Women's HealthSource* article, "Food Cravings: Shaking the Salt Habit," recommends replacing salt with herbs and spices.

The article gives some conversion ratios. For example, 1 tablespoon of a fresh herb equals H teaspoon of a dry herb. With the exception of basil (I'm a basil nut) I follow this formula. I crush dry herbs with my fingers to bring out the flavor before adding them to recipes.

Herbs and spices should be stored in airtight containers. Cookbooks advise discarding herbs and spices that are more than a year old. For this reason, I never buy herbs and spices in jumbo sizes.

Manufacturers are developing new products, such as garlic pepper, Jane's Krazy Mixed-Up Pepper, and Mrs. Dash products, to meet consumer needs. Schilling has come out with an All-Purpose Table Shake Seasoning. I often add citrus zest to recipes to boost flavor.

An article in the *Journal of the American Medical Association* also advises cutting down on salt. Dietary intervention was the focus of the study, "Sodium Reduction and Weight Loss in the Treatment of Hypertension in Older Persons," by Paul Whelton, MD, MSc, and his colleagues.

Knowledge about diet and behavior were the main goals of the study. The researchers studied 585 obese patients, 60 to 80 years old, who had been diagnosed with high blood pressure. A variety of interventions were set up for the patients, including diet modification, problem-solving, and relapse prevention. "Withdrawal of antihypertensive medication was a goal for all study participants," note the researchers. They found that reducing salt and weight resulted in lower blood pressure. The researchers say there is a need for sodium-reduced processed foods. Certainly, my husband and I found this to be true.

Cut the Fat

Most Americans eat a high-fat diet, according to dietitian
Ronni Chernoff, PhD, RD. Fat is just one of the topics she
addresses in her study, "Effect of Age on Nutrient Requirements." About 10 percent of our food intake should come
from unsaturated fat, Chernoff explains, but the American
diet is approximately 40 percent fat. What a difference!

No wonder doctors are urging their patients to cut the fat.
You can still eat the foods you enjoy, even foods you crave,
but in moderation. I checked frozen pizza labels and found
that one slice of pepperoni pizza contained 12 fat grams and
30 milligrams of cholesterol. So-called "light" pizza wasn't
much better. One-fifth of a light vegetable pizza contained 7
grams of fat and 10 milligrams of cholesterol.

You may have to become a kitchen chemist to cut the fat.
After experimenting with many recipes (some successful,
some disastrous) I cut fat automatically. I replace half the
shortening in baked goods with sugar-free applesauce. Instead of eggs, I use a noncholesterol egg white product.

Good pans are essential to cutting the fat; I have nonstick
skillets in various sizes. My newest kitchen treasure is a cast
iron grill pan. Unlike the nonstick skillets, I can preheat this
pan until it is smoking hot, and sear food quickly. Cast iron
pans will last a lifetime if you follow the manufacturer's seasoning and washing directions.

Increase Fiber

Americans are buying more convenience foods than ever
before, including food kits, sauce mixes, frozen dinners, and
take-out. These foods are often high in fat and salt, and low
in fiber. If you rely on mixes and take-out, find ways to add
fiber to your meal. Eat an apple, some peas, a spinach salad,
or a slice of whole wheat bread.

My homemade oatmeal bread with walnuts is a family favorite. This bread tastes good with everything: salads, pasta,

stir-fry, you name it. Oats, oat bran, and other fiber help to keep bowels regular, help irritable bowel syndrome, and may lower your risk of colon cancer.

Drink Water

Water is an essential nutrient for aging people; it's crucial to life. About 56 percent of the human body is water and we need to stay hydrated. Lack of fluid can have serious effects, according to Ronni Chernoff, PhD, RD, author of "Effects of Age on Nutrient Requirements," including:

- rapid dehydration
- low blood pressure (hypotension)
- fever
- constipation
- nausea
- vomiting
- nose/mouth dryness
- decreased urine output
- general confusion

Dehydration is one of the topics Jean Merhinge Winger and Thomas Hornick cover in their study, "Age Associated Changes in the Endocrine System." They say aging people get dehydrated because of impaired thirst perception, failure to recognize/respond to water deprivation, and greater risk of dehydration. We may be dehydrated and not know it.

Reading about dehydration made me realize that I needed to drink more water. To ensure proper hydration, I drink a glass of water with each meal. In the mid-afternoon I drink another glass of water. As my mother used to say, "There's nothing wrong with Adam's ale." Healthy eating should be combined with an exercise program.

Exercise

Why should you exercise? Zebulon Kendrick, PhD, and his colleagues tell why in their study, "Metabolic and Nutritional Considerations for Exercising Older Adults."

They use statistics to make the exercise case and the numbers got my attention. A 1985 National Health Promotion Interview survey found that a mere 7.5 percent of Americans 65 years old and older participated in aerobic activity. A 1990 Public Health Service survey found that only 50 percent of Americans 65 years old and older engaged in any physical activity at all.

Misconceptions about exercise may cause us to ignore it. You may think you need less exercise as you age or convince yourself that occasional exercise is as beneficial as regular exercise. Lack of exercise may be due to physical problems. Your doctor will be able to tell you which type of exercise suits you best. Just a few stretches a day can be beneficial. Competitive sports are not for me. However, I discovered, like other aging people, that exercise makes me feel better.

Ilkka Vuori emphasizes the importance of exercise in his study, "Exercise and Physical Health: Musculoskeletal Health and Functional Capabilities." The Finnish researcher says bone mineral density starts to decline when we are in our early 30s. But something else is going on. "A substantial part of the age-related decline in functional capabilities is not due to aging per se but due to decreased and insufficient physical activity." In short, we have to keep moving.

The exercise theme isn't just for the "old folks." Whenever I go to a shopping mall I am shocked at the size of today's teens. Not only are they taller than my generation, many seem to be overweight and in poor condition. I watched a teen run to catch up with his friends and he was out of breath in a few steps.

Henry Barry, MD, and Scott Eathorne, MD, take a close

look at exercise in their study, "Exercise and Aging: Issues for the Practitioner." Physical inactivity may put us at risk for diseases such as coronary artery disease, osteoporosis, obesity, and diabetes, say the researchers.

Get a pre-exercise evaluation before you start an exercise program. The evaluation should include "goal identification, evaluation of medical history and physical examination, and assessing fitness level," according to Barry and Eathorne. They recommend a five-point program.

1. Consistent energy expenditure

2. Specific duration

3. Frequency

4. Pursuit of fitness goals

5. Your progress

"The length a given activity is performed should be inversely related to the intensity of the activity," they explain. Aging people should drink fluids before exercising and take scheduled water breaks. Layer your clothing so you can adjust to temperature changes. Track your progress in an exercise diary.

Make Exercise Fun

Seniors are getting the exercise message. An Associated Press article, "Seniors Seeking Friends and Fitness on a Roll With Skating," tells about seniors who roller skate weekly. The sessions began at the World of Wheels in Superior, Wisconsin, in the 1940s. "Everybody knows everybody," Beverly Kallberg is quoted as saying.

The skaters enjoy the musical selections, the freedom of skating, and its exercise benefits. One member of the group said skating kept him fit for skiing. While roller skating may not be your first exercise choice, you can still exercise. You might want to start by investing in some indoor equipment.

Television infomercials show young people doing weird things with muffler pipe. The stars of these commercials are so perky you could throw up. What's more, their bodies bend and stretch like rubber bands. They sit on the pipe, lie beneath it, and move it in various directions, all the while smiling into the camera.

Of course these people look fit; they are decades younger than I. Does the equipment help them? It's hard to say without knowing how many hours a day they exercise.

Do some comparison shopping before you buy any indoor equipment. You may choose weights, a stationary bike, rowing machine, treadmill, stair climber, or cross country ski machine.

"Exercise Equipment," an article in the *Mayo Clinic Health Letter*, lists some points to consider:

1. Construction of the equipment

2. Fit and feel

3. Is there a free trial period?

4. Do free instructions come with the equipment?

5. Are any "extras" included?

6. What are the terms of the guarantee or warranty?

I exercise on a 25-year-old Schwinn stationary bike (almost a museum piece) that came with a lifetime guarantee. Schwinn stood by this guarantee and gave me new pedal straps when the old ones wore out. Where you exercise has a lot to do with how often you use the equipment.

Our house is below the rim of a hill. I used to exercise in my basement office, which had no television reception and scratchy radio reception. Needless to say, I didn't exercise very much. Now that the bike is in the family room in front of cable TV I use it daily.

Check newspaper ads for used equipment. Our weekly

shopping paper had three ads in one issue and they used similar language: "never used," "barely used," "like new." You may be able to get top-notch equipment at a bargain price. Work up to your exercise rate gradually.

Men who bike for long periods of time should use caution. A Norwegian study by Kjeld Andersen and Gunnar Bovim, "Impotence and Nerve Entrapment in Long Distance Amateur Cyclists," reports excessive biking may lead to penis numbness, hand weakness, and finger problems. These findings were based on a survey of 260 bikers who completed a 540 kilometer amateur touring race from Trondheim to Oslo, known as "The Great Trial of Strength."

A whole body drawing was sent to the bikers along with the questionnaire. The bikers were asked to color in pain, numbness, and parathesia areas (often called pins and needles) on the drawing. After completing the race, 21 males reported impotence.

Eleven of these men said the impotence lasted at least a week. Two men, ages 31 and 42, said it lasted for months. "The mechanism of impotence caused by nerve compression is not readily understood," say the researchers. They suggest changing hand/body position, restricting exercise, and taking breaks to prevent impotence and nerve damage.

Other cases of bike-induced impotence appear in the medical literature. In some cases, doctors were able to reverse temporary impotence, but other men were not as fortunate.

Pamper Your Feet

Taking care of your feet is another step on the road to successful aging. Arthur Helfand, DPM, discusses foot care in his study, "Assessment of the Geriatric Patient." He believes one of the main goals of health professionals is to keep their patients walking. This goal "needs to be met if older persons are to maintain a high degree of quality in their lives."

Feet are subjected to normal use, misuse, trauma, and neglect. The condition of our feet depends on past work, activity level, weight, disease (such as diabetes), and vein problems. Doctors can learn a lot about you just by examining your feet. Cold feet may be an indication of poor circulation. Foot drop may be an indication of neurological damage. Swollen feet may be an indication of heart problems. Be sure to tell your doctor about any foot problems you may have.

Also make sure you are wearing the right size shoes. Women's feet grow one size for every child they have, according to an old wives' tale, and it has been true for me. This may be a good time to get your feet measured if you haven't done it recently. Choose a reliable shoe store and a reliable sales associate.

Get Enough Sleep

Physical changes may prevent us from getting enough sleep. Martin Gorbein, MD, detailed some of the changes in his study, "When Your Older Patient Can't Sleep: How to Put Insomnia to Rest." Gorbein, who heads the Geriatric Medicine, Department of Internal Medicine at the Cleveland Clinic, says women have more sleep complaints than men.

Older people wake up more often than younger people. We are also less adaptable to changes in our sleep conditions, such as a strange bed, too much light, and temperature changes. Gorbein explains that physical problems encompass a broad range:

- Shortness of breath
- Leg cramps
- More bathroom stops (nocturia)
- Thyroid dysfunction
- Chest and stomach pain
- Medications (diet pills, meds that contain caffeine)

The medical and psychiatric causes of poor sleep often overlap. "Patients with depression typically report early morning arousal with an inability to fall back to sleep," explains Gorbein. Aging people who are depressed may suffer from a variety of sleep disorders.

Two Ohio researchers, Michael Bonnet, PhD, and Donna Arand think many of us are sleep deprived. Their study, "We Are Chronically Sleep Deprived," attributes sleep loss to fragmented sleep. The researchers estimate that 7 percent of the middle-aged people in our country are "excessively sleepy."

News headlines list sleep deprivation as the cause of plane, train, and car crashes. According to the researchers, the cost of sleep-related accidents in the United States ranges from 2 to 56 billion dollars per year. The solution: more sleep and better sleep. "Studies have already shown significantly improved performance and alertness when time in bed is increased from 8 to 10 hours per night," say the researchers.

Sleep Disorders

Aging people who have a sleep disorder find it hard to get any sleep at all. Dr. Patricia Prinz focuses on sleep disorders in her study, "Sleep and Sleep Disorders in Older Adults." She believes circadian rhythm problems keep some of us awake. If you have flown halfway around the world, and come home totally exhausted, you may not be able to fall asleep.

Restless legs, the urge to repeatedly move your legs before falling asleep, may keep you awake. The causes of restless legs are unknown. Some of us are restless and awake because we are in pain. Arthritis, varicose veins, and sore feet may cause us to move about. You may find it hard to find a comfortable sleeping position.

Buy a foam topper for your mattress if you are uncomfortable. Forego sleep during the day to promote sleep at night. If you feel you need a nap, don't sleep for more than a half hour. Limit your caffeine and alcohol consumption.

Exercise regularly, but don't do anything strenuous before bedtime. Don't take a hot shower or bath before bedtime because that could keep you awake as well.

Sleeping aids should be used cautiously, according to Dr. Martin Gorbein. "Despite the many studies illustrating the safety of sedative/hypnotics in older patients, the incidence of adverse effects rises with increased age and dosage," he writes. Talk with your doctor before you take any sleeping aids.

Track Your Meds

As we get older we may take more medicine. First one pill, then two, then more. Problems arise when the medicines interact unfavorably with each other. So track the medicine you are taking and be aware of drug interactions. A *Family Circle* magazine insert by Ilene Springer, "Health Alert! Drugs That Don't Mix," gives readers an overview of drug interactions.

The chart has four headings: Brand Name/Generic, Purpose, Use Caution if Also Taking, and Possible Effects if Combined. It shows that Tums (calcium carbonate) should not be taken with tetracycline, for example. Calcium carbonate decreases the effectiveness of tetracycline.

Be cautious of products that are sold as food supplements. The Food and Drug Administration (FDA) does not review food supplements the same way it reviews drugs. You may have allergic or toxic reactions to the supplements. Food supplements may also alter the effects of any prescribed medication you are taking.

Berry Kendler, PhD, takes a critical look at one food supplement in his study, "Melatonin: Media Hype or Therapeutic Breakthrough?" Melatonin is made from an essential amino acid (tryptophan) and is used to treat jet lag, delayed sleep, sleep disorders, and even cancer. When samples were obtained from health food stores, however, four out of six contained what Kendler calls "unidentifiable impurities." Other researchers are expressing concern about melatonin.

According to Billie Holliman, PharmD, and Peter Chyka, PharmD, authors of "Problems in Assessment of Acute Melatonin Overdose," there is insufficient data about the product. They write, "Questions about proper dose, interactions with other drugs, and long-term effectiveness and safety remain unanswered."

After revising food labels in 1993 the FDA also revised supplement labels. The standarized labels must list the contents, dosage, and added ingredients. A disclaimer was added to the labels: "This product is not intended to diagnose, treat, cure, or prevent any disease." However, the manufacturers are allowed to make general health claims, such as "improve urine flow."

The labels have given some consumers a false sense of security. Medical writer Jane Brody expresses her concerns in her article, "Supplement Use is Unregulated Minefield." Since the FDA doesn't require manufacturers to conduct clinical trials, Brody thinks consumers may be, "in effect, serving as guinea pigs in experiments that don't always have happy endings."

The FDA doesn't require manufacturers to prove their advertising claims either. A standardized label is of little use if you don't know what is in the bottle. Mel Borins, MD, in his study "The Dangers of Using Herbs," says supplements have been contaminated with arsenic, mercury, and lead. Commonly used herbs can have serious side effects, including hypertension, irregular heart beats, abnormal bleeding, liver damage, and hepatitis.

"Herbal Roulette," an article published in *Consumer Re-*

ports, says consumers have many questions to answer:

- Is the label wording true?
- Have other ingredients (not listed on the label) been added to the product?
- Is the supplement in a form your body can use?
- Is the product safe?
- Does the manufacturer have quality control?
- Has the product been standardized?

Cost is another factor to consider. As many consumers have discovered, the yearly cost of food supplements adds up quickly. One patient admitted to spending hundreds of dollars on the 30-some supplements he was taking. "I suspect he was taking more than that," said his doctor.

An estimated one out of every three Americans is taking a food supplement. Many don't tell their doctors about the supplements, which distorts medical tests, and ultimately, medical diagnosis. Some consumers take "natural" supplements because they assume natural means safe.

It's a dangerous assumption, says toxicologist Mary Palmer, MD, in her study, "Dietary Supplements: 'Natural' is not Always Safe." The word supplement can means plants, herbs, blue-green algae, vitamins, minerals, hormones, amino acids, and cultural remedies, explains Palmer. "Not only are dietary supplements poorly studied and unregulated, but reliable records of adverse effects are sadly lacking."

In short, this is a buyer beware market. Remember, aging people react differently to medication than younger people. Before you follow a food fad, whether it's ginko biloba, fen phen, or garlic, talk with your doctor. Tell your doctor about any supplements you may be taking. For more information contact:

- MEDWATCH at 800-FDA-4010

- NAPRALERT (Natural Products Alert program sponsored by the University of Illinois) at 312-996-2246
- Centers for Disease Control, Dr. Roffane Philen, at 770-488-7350
- MEDLINE data base at www.ncbi.nlm.nih.gov/pubmed
- American Botanical Council at www.herbalgram.org

Regular Dental Care

Dental checkups reveal cavities, gum disease, receding gums, cracked teeth, and other oral hygiene problems. A variety of barriers prevent aging people from getting regular dental care. Cost is a major barrier for some. Often insurance plans cover partial care, not all, and a visit to the dentist is postponed.

Studies show that aging people are also afraid to go to the dentist. The result isn't just poor oral hygiene, it may be disease that endangers your health. Douglas Berkey, DMD, MPH, MS, makes this point in his editorial, "Geriatric Dentistry at the Crossroads." Chair of the Department of Dentistry at the University of Colorado School of Dentistry, Berkey thinks dental schools need to emphasize the link between oral and general health. Improving the health of at risk populations and care of the aging should also be emphasized.

COMPOSITE MATERIALS

My dentist says the two hottest trends in dentistry today are geriatrics and composite materials. He told me this as he was installing a crown on my tooth with fast-acting glue. The glue felt hot at first and then cooled quickly. "This will never come off," he assured me.

The St. Paul-based 3M company is one of the major manufacturers of dental materials. An article in the company newsletter, "3M Employees Gather to Celebrate Dental Products' Achievement," says the Dental Products Division makes more than 700 different products, used by dentists world-wide.

Composite engineers continue to invent new dental materials. What is a composite? The *ASM International Manual* (the initials stand for the American Society for Metals) defines a composite as a combination of two or more materials. These materials—reinforcing elements, fillers, and matrix binders—work in concert with one another. The materials retain their separate identities and can still be identified.

Plastic sealants, either clear or shaded, are another trend in dentistry. According to "Seal Out Decay," an American Dental Association brochure, the sealant is applied to the chewing surface of the back teeth. Sealants have been around for a long time, but many patients are just discovering them. Kids derive the greatest benefit from sealants, and one application can last for years.

FLUORIDE

Whether it is in the water you drink or the toothpaste you use, fluoride continues to be important in dentistry. Dentists say we shouldn't be fooled by toothpastes that foam. The foaming action gives some people a false sense of security. Instead of brushing thoroughly, they do a token job, and think the foaming action is doing the rest.

Dentists are impressed by a new anti-cavity fluoride toothpaste, called Enamelon, that strengthens tooth enamel. This toothpaste can be especially helpful to the aging, whose teeth are beginning to show signs of wear. Regular dental care can help your teeth to last a lifetime.

Laser Surgery

Lasers are used to treat acne rosacea and detaching retina, among other things. Diane Thiboutot, MD, of the Pennsylvania State University College of Medicine, focuses on the laser treatment of acne in her study, "Acne Rosacea." Vascular skin lesions may respond to treatment that involves the use of something called a tunable dye laser. "When tuned to the wavelength at which blood vessels absorb light, effective treatment of vascular lesions can be accomplished with little scarring or damage to surrounding skin," she writes.

Lasers have been used to treat gross deformities of the nose. Thiboutot says the idea is to restore the nose to a normal shape with minimal scarring.

 As I discovered, lasers are being used to treat detaching retinas. Despite a friend's detailed account of her symptoms and surgery, I did not realize I had a detaching retina until I went to the eye doctor. However, I had been concerned enough about my symptoms—eye floaters that looked like insects and lightning flashes—to make an appointment.

I was given two kinds of eye drops, one to dilate my eye, the other to anesthetize it. The eye doctor gave me a thorough exam. "You have a detaching retina," she announced. "We'll have it fixed in 15 minutes."

She turned on the laser machine (it hummed a little) and put the beam up to my eye. It was the brightest light I had ever seen, so intense I wondered if I could withstand it.

Still, I knew I was in good hands. Carefully and systematically, the doctor "welded" my detaching retina together.

"This is going very well," she said, turning the laser at a 45 degree angle. The surgery did not correct my vision problem, but it did keep my vision from getting any worse. Interestingly, my brother had the same surgery in his right eye. Doctors think this is a coincidence and not a genetic defect.

Chemical Peels/Dermabrasion

Henry Roenigk, MD, details laser surgery in his study, "The Place of Laser Resurfacing Within the Range of Medical and Surgical Skin Resurfacing Techniques." He thinks chemical peels are a safe way to remove wrinkles on aging hands and faces.

Dermabrasion is another type of treatment and, according to Roenigk, "the results in areas such as the forehead or perioral area are comparable to laser resurfacing." Doctors may combine a chemical peel with dermabrasion. Laser resurfacing is ideal for crow's feet and fine wrinkles on the eyelids. "Do what is best for the patient," Roenigk advises.

Plastic Surgery

Thanks to computer technology, doctors can predict how you will look after plastic surgery. Associated Press writer Malcom Ritter gives an update on plastic surgery in his article, "Fix Your Face: More and More Men Removing Bags, Sags." Ritter says the American Society of Plastic and Reconstructive Surgeons did 5,000 facelifts on men in 1996.

"The society counted about 11,200 male patients for eyelid procedure last year, up about 25 percent," he writes. Men are having facelifts, browlifts, chin liposuction, and laser treatment for spider veins and creases. Why are the numbers going up?

Ritter thinks it's because men want to look better at work and have a competitive edge. But plastic surgery is major surgery and we need to remember that. Choose a board-certified doctor if you are thinking about having plastic surgery.

Laura Fraser writes about an unreliable surgeon in her magazine article, "The Case of the Dangerous Doctor." She tells the story of San Francisco plastic surgeon Allyn Beth Landau, MD, who used slick advertising to lure patients. Landau's newspaper ads listed impressive credentials and promised to help with wrinkles, acne scars, lip augmentation, "fresh eyes," complexion rejuvenation, and more. One patient, who sought advice for 10 moles on her arm, saw her only once. The surgical removal of the moles was done by an assistant. However, the patient felt uneasy and saw another doctor.

It turns out she had skin cancer. The cancerous tissue, along with some lymph nodes, were surgically removed and she is cancer-free today. Eventually the California Medical Board revoked Landau's license for failure to notify patients about their pathology reports and for using untrained staff. Dr. Landau is appealing the case.

Clearly, plastic surgery has helped many people to overcome disfigurements and the effects of aging. To find a board-certified plastic surgeon call the American Society for Dermatologic Surgery at 1-800-441-2737.

Vein Therapy

In the last few years the treatments for varicose veins have improved. The treatments are effective and quick, some taking less than an hour. "Varicose Veins," an article in the *Mayo Clinic Women's HealthSource,* discusses three treatments: sclerotherapy, ambulatory phlebectomy, and laser.

With sclerotherapy, a solution is injected into the varicose vein to chemically destroy it. The procedure requires no anesthesia but may require several treatments. Bruising and skin discoloration are two side effects of treatment.

For ambulatory phlebectomy, tiny punctures are made on the skin's surface and varicose veins are pulled through them. The procedure is done under local anesthesia. There is little skin discoloration and scarring.

So-called spider veins may be removed with an intense pulsed light or laser. The procedure causes the veins to shrink, collapse, and disappear. Some changes in skin pigmentation may result from these procedures, so take this into account before you agree to surgery.

Stop Smoking

One of the best things you can do to age successfully is to stop smoking. The medical evidence on the dangers of tobacco can no longer be ignored. Whatever the form—cigarettes, cigars, or chewing tobacco—tobacco is harmful. Just a few facts:

- Tobacco contains 4,000 chemical compounds, including carbon monoxide.
- Nicotine in tobacco increases the body's heart rate and blood pressure.
- Long-term use of tobacco damages the lungs.
- Tobacco alters the clotting properties of blood.
- Tobacco causes a decrease in the body's high density lipoprotein ("good cholesterol")
- Some doctors think tobacco smoke damages hearing.
- People who use chewing tobacco run the risk of developing mouth cancer.

The death certificate lists pneumonia as the cause of my father's death, but I know tobacco killed him. He smoked at least two packs of cigarettes a day. The cigarette smell permeated the house and my eyes were hypersensitive to the smoke. If I was anywhere near Dad my eyelids would swell until they were slits on my face. Sometimes my eyes swelled shut. That didn't stop Dad from sitting in his brown leather chair, staring into space, and smoking one cigarette after another. The price of cigarettes kept going up so Dad bought a cigarette machine. When I was in grade school I was intrigued by the machine's roller mechanism. I grew to hate the machine and the habit it served.

Dad smoked through my college years, my early marriage years, and my daughters' high school years, until he needed oxygen to breathe. His lungs were so damaged that Dad couldn't walk three feet from the front door to the mailbox.

An oxygen tank became his constant companion.

Finally, Dad was hospitalized for emphysema and I flew home to see him. Glad as he was to see me, Dad was very grouchy, and I mentioned this to his nurse. "You'd be grouchy, too, if you thought each breath was your last," she commented. I have thought of her reply many times.

The time came when my father's medical needs exceeded my mother's capacity to care for him. With help from the fire department, she got him into a firemen's home in up-state New York, where he died at age 80. His terrible, tortuous death changed me forever. I get upset when I see kids smoking and want to rush up to them and say, "Stop! You're killing yourself!"

Use a Support System

Experts say we age more successfully if we have a support system. Being part of a group is an empowering experience, according to researchers Renee Solomon, DSW, and Monte Peterson, MD. Their study, "Successful Aging: How to Help Your Patients Cope With Change," says three services are essential: access to health care, safe housing, and medical/welfare benefits.

You may have some or all of these services, depending on where you have worked and where you live. Social workers will be glad to connect you with the help you need. Age may determine your support system and how often you use it.

Raymond Bossé and his colleagues make this point in their study, "Change in Social Support After Retirement: Longitudinal Findings from the Normative Aging Study."

Their study builds on a previous study conducted by the Veterans Administration. Questionnaires were sent to veterans about changes in the quality and quantity of support. A total of 1,311 veterans participated in the study.

The researchers were surprised to learn that quantitative

support (number of times used) declined equally for all groups. The worsening economy between 1985 and 1988 may have caused the respondents to socialize less. Answering the same questions twice in a three year time span may have also influenced results.

Still, the researchers were encouraged by their findings. "Although one may lose family and friends so that the social support network declines, the quality or the perception of support available did not decline over time and did not differ between long-term retirees and men who continued to work."

Support is essential if you use a home health care system. That is one message in "Social Support and the Elderly Client," by Esther Hellman, MS, RN, and Cynthia Stewart, PhD, RN. The researchers studied 57 clients who had been discharged from "a Midwestern, multi-office, nonprofit home healthcare agency." Clients were 65 years old or older, had received at least two home visits, were released to family care, and were mentally alert.

Ninety-five percent of the clients received some kind of support, either from children, relatives, friends, or neighbors. One-third of the clients (32 percent) said they needed more help with nursing care, housework, fixing meals, rides to medical care, and shopping. In other words, their support systems were inadequate.

You probably have a support system. Does it meet your needs? Take a close look at your support system and make any necessary changes. While you are doing this, you might offer to help someone else. A brief meeting or phone call can change someone's life.

So you see, there are steps you can take to age successfully. Your steps add up over time. One other step, understanding sexuality in the aging, has been omitted from this chapter. This step is so important it has a chapter of its own, "Sexuality, Intimacy, and Love," which comes next.

Smart Aging Tips

- Eat right.
- Get enough calcium.
- Hold the salt.
- Cut the fat.
- Add more fiber to your diet.
- Drink enough water.
- Exercise regularly.
- Pamper your feet.
- Get enough sleep.
- Track the medicine you take.
- Visit the dentist regularly.
- Ask your doctor about laser surgery, chemical peels, dermabrasion, or plastic surgery.
- Learn more about vein therapy.
- If you are still smoking, stop.
- Use a support system.

5

Sexuality, Intimacy, and Love

"*The publisher wants me* to tell personal stories," I told my husband at dinnertime. "I'm trying to include at least two stories in each chapter."

"What chapter are you working on now?" he asked.

"Sexuality and intimacy."

My husband almost dropped his fork. "You're not going to..."

"No, I'm not going to tell stories about our sex life," I assured him. "But I am going to tell some things about our relationship."

"That's OK" he said, and we immediately got into a conversation about our marriage. Friends often comment on what a loving couple we are and this makes us feel good. We think we know why our marriage works, but we aren't sure, and have decided not to overanalyze it.

I think we have a good marriage because we knew each other well before we married. We listen to each other and this has led to mutual respect. Forty-one years together haven't eliminated the element of surprise from our marriage. We make each other laugh. Best of all, we know we can always count on one another. My husband is my champion and I am his.

Sexuality is part of our lives. Younger people may not believe this, however, because they don't know much about sexuality in the aging. Our society seems to think young people are the only ones with sexual feelings. And sexuality is, by itself, a complex topic.

Fran Kaiser, MD, author of "Sexuality in the Elderly," thinks the topic covers attitudes, behavior, practices, and activity. Many people believe that loss of sexuality comes with age and this belief is false. Sexuality is part of the human condition and continues throughout life. It is nature's way of ensuring the survival of the species.

Sexuality Is Cumulative

There is no age at which thoughts about sexuality and sexual activity end, according to Kaiser. Experts say our past experience influences future sexual behavior. If you have a passionate relationship in your younger years, chances are you will have a similar sexual relationship in your later years. As Kaiser writes, "Another 'predictor' [of sexuality] appears to be sexual interest, enjoyment, and activity in younger years."

The mind is the body's main sexual organ. When I look at my husband I see a man approaching retirement age. I also see a man who was a James Dean look-alike in his youth, a man who bought me gifts on his birthday, the Air Force officer who received the Bronze Star for valor in Vietnam, a loving father to our daughters, a dedicated health professional, and a sweet grandfather who plays games with the twins. I see the experiences that made the man.

My husband has a similar reaction when he looks at me. He sees the 17-year-old woman he met two weeks after starting college, a person who loves to learn, a competent cook, a community volunteer, an amateur decorator, an adoring grandmother, and a nonfiction writer.

We see each other through the colorful, changing kaleidoscope of life experience. Time has increased the sexual excitement we feel for one another. Being with my husband makes me feel 17 again. Despite our respective health scares, we are in pretty good health, thanks to modern medicine. We have been blessed. But health is a barrier to sexuality for many aging people.

Barriers to Sexuality

Diana Wiley and Walter Bortz II studied sexuality and report their findings in "Sexuality and Aging—Usual and Successful." They began their study with a three-part series on sexuality at the Palo Alto, California, Senior Center. An average of 58 people attended the series.

Wiley and Bortz surveyed the attendees to get some personal information on sexuality. Six months later they sent a follow-up questionnaire to the attendees. The questionnaire topics included the importance of kissing, oral sex, manual genital stimulation, sexual intercourse, orgasm, loving and caring, and satisfying your partner.

Current findings were compared to past findings. Wiley and Bortz say their current findings about sexual enjoyment are more complex than the ones gathered 10 years ago.

- Roughly 32 percent said the frequency of sexual activity had not changed in 10 years
- 60 percent reported a decrease in sexual activity
- 8 percent reported an increase in sexual activity
- More males (71 percent) wanted increased sexual activity
- 52 percent of females said they wanted an increase
- About 50 percent of both males and females said they thought less about sex now as compared to a decade ago

"Whereas our follow-up questionnaire showed no real

change in sexual behaviors, there was a substantial expression of increased knowledge, confidence, and sensitivity," the researchers write.

Illness, relationship problems, and erection difficulties were some of the causes of decreased sexual activity. The death of a spouse may close the door on the known sexuality of the past and open the door to sexual exploration. Older women who don't have a male partner or the prospect of one may express their sexuality with other women.

In her book, *Be An Outrageous Older Woman,* Ruth Harriet Jacobs, PhD, says this expression of sexuality may be overt or sublimated. She lists some of the ways older women may express sexuality: intercourse with a husband, vacationing with male friends, self-pleasure, reading sexual novels, seeing sexual movies, joining singles groups, focusing attention on children and grandchildren, choosing celibacy, and marrying again.

Lesbians may look for another lesbian partner after a partner dies. Jacobs says lifelong lesbians face the same kind of sexual deprivations as heterosexual women. "Maybe I have shocked you with my frank chapter," she writes. "But I could back it up by references in the scientific literature."

Medication, environment, and chronic illness are also barriers to sexuality in the aging. For some, living in a nursing home is a sexual barrier. Further complicating the issue is the fact that many nursing home employees have little or no sexuality training.

Chronic illness, financial problems, and the vulnerability of age force some parents to move in with their adult children. This arrangement tests the old and the young. Living with children can put a damper on the parent's sexuality and their children's as well.

Increasingly, grown children are moving back home to regroup. The timing is poor. Just when parents have gotten used to their honeymoon nest, they have adult children underfoot, and the hassles that come with it. "He's up watching TV half the night," a father complained. "We can't sleep, let alone have sex."

Life-threatening illness is another barrier to sexuality. Let's say one partner has a heart defect that requires surgery. The surgery is successful and the patient is restored to good health. Long after surgery, however, the fear of relapse is still present. This mental barrier may alter sexual behavior.

The Sexuality/Health Equation

Stephen Holzapfel, MD, CCFP, of the Department of Family and Community Medicine at the University of Toronto Medical School, studies sexuality in the aging population. He views sexual expression in the aging as a predictor of general health. In other words, people who have good health continue to be sexual. "The greatest barrier to being sexual in old age is lack of a healthy sexual partner," he writes in his study "Aging and Sexuality."

Menopause affects sexuality in older females. Women spend about a third of their lives in menopause, according to Holzapfel, and that is a large chunk of time. Medication may also alter our sexual performance. People who are 65 years old and above take roughly three times as many prescription drugs as younger people. Holzapfel notes that medical treatment—medicine, surgery, rehabilitation—is the most common cause of sexual dysfunction.

Many doctors are reluctant to bring up the topic of sexuality with their patients because it is embarrassing. Whether we are embarrassed or not, aging people are sexual people, and that is a fact. The sexuality equation has many components and they may, or may not, balance. Society's view of sexuality is one of these components.

"I'm Sexually Invisible."

When I told a friend of mine that I was going to write a book about aging, she immediately asked, "What's in it?" I listed some of the topics, including sexuality, and she interrupted me. "That's good, because I'm sexually invisible," she said. "Nobody thinks I am a sexual person anymore. It's awful."

Once you are sexually invisible you may also become generally invisible. Sexual invisibility is like a leaking faucet; it begins with one drip, or one experience. More experiences come, faster and faster, until there is a constant stream of sexual invisibility. You may be ignored while standing in line, for example, or patronized by younger co-workers.

A recent trip to the drive-in bank made me feel totally invisible. I wrote a check for 75 dollars, put it in the tube, and sent the tube to the teller. The tube came back empty, so I pressed the service button. Nothing happened. I pressed the service button again and, still, nothing happened. Although I could see the teller, somehow she couldn't see me.

In desperation, I started waving at the teller. The intercom came on with a crackling sound. "May I help you?" she asked in an annoyed voice.

"Yes, you can give me my money," I said. "I wrote a check for 75 dollars and the tube came back empty."

The teller was startled. "Just a minute," she answered. A few minutes later the tube came back with 75 dollars in it. "Sorry about that," she said. "I didn't think anyone was there."

Didn't think anyone was there? I was sitting in a red car, pressing the service button repeatedly, waving at the teller, and she didn't think anyone was there? Her apology was vexing. Age discrimination is the real issue here, society's way of saying we aren't worth noticing.

Unlike the Oriental cultures, which respect age, our society views the aging as dried up, useless, sexless people.

At home I am a cherished wife. My husband and I show affection in front of the twins so they know their grandparents love each other. The twins are getting the idea. We were playing a self-esteem game with them and my husband's game piece landed on a square that read, "Say something nice about the person next to you."

He gave me a hug, and said, "You are beautiful."

Our granddaughter beamed. A few minutes later, her game piece landed on a square that asked her to list something that made her happy. Her reply: "When people say I'm beautiful."

"And you are beautiful," I added.

Some day, and it will probably come sooner than I expect, the twins will figure out that we are sexual people. Until that time comes, they know love is the cornerstone of our family, our love for each other, our love for our children, and our love for them.

Sexual Dysfunction in Men

Two major problems, erectile dysfunction and Widower's Syndrome, prevent many men from expressing their sexuality. The causes of erectile dysfunction include vascular disorders, medication (such as diuretics and hypertensives), tobacco, marijuana, alcohol, neurologic disorders, and psychological problems.

Widower's Syndrome "may result from unresolved guilt and grief toward the deceased partner, and subconscious repression of sexual feelings," according to Fran Kaiser, MD. Painful memories may also contribute to Widower's Syndrome. Grief is a process that takes time. Sadly, time may not heal this wound.

Sexual Dysfunction in Women

Women who have difficult or painful intercourse may become sexually dysfunctional. Sex becomes something to fear, rather than a joyous celebration of life. Lack of vaginal lubrication may also make intercourse painful. Incontinence may also inhibit sexual desire, according to Kaiser.

Hysterectomy, which has been performed on one-third of the women in our country over age 60, is not associated with sexual dysfunction. However, Kaiser says the women who associate a hysterectomy with loss of femininity may experience some problems.

Vaginismus (painful spasms of the vaginal muscles) may also contribute to sexual dysfunction. Yeast infections, which are fairly common in aging women, also play a part in sexual displeasure. As you might expect, menopause has a profound effect on female sexuality.

Menopause

The treatment for menopause continues to improve. Gloria Bachmann, MD, describes treatment in her study, "Influence of Menopause on Sexuality." Hormone replacement therapy (HRT) is one focus of her study. As she writes, "The importance of hormone replacement therapy in four areas of menopausal health is quite clear: cardiovascular health, prevention of osteoporosis, control of vasomotor symptoms, and maintenance of urogenital health."

Bachmann discusses the effects of decreased estrogen levels on sexual function and they are considerable:

- Decreased support of pelvis (which affects sexual satisfaction)
- Loss of lubrication (which may make intercourse painful)
- Changes in body configuration
- Skin changes (touch may be less pleasurable)
- Breast changes
- Muscular and skeletal loss

Many people assume males are always "sexually ready" and this isn't true. Bachmann says the male partner may have less sexual interest and this leads to a decline in sexual activity. In contrast, women who have completed menopause may feel sexually freer because they no longer worry about getting pregnant.

Hormone replacement therapy has been part of my life for more than 15 years. Migraine headaches are a side-effect of this therapy. Although I don't have full-blown migraines, I have colorful auras —displays of zig-zag lines and flashing lights. The auras can hit at the worst times.

I was on the way to a conference in St. Paul when an aura developed. It got progressively worse and by the time I reached the city my field of vision had been reduced to a circle. Traffic was heavy and I couldn't find a place to pull over. Since I was two blocks from my destination, I slowed down, continued on to the hotel, and arrived safely.

But my circle of vision got even smaller, and I was having trouble thinking. I went to the ladies room before the meeting started. As I was washing my hands I realized the ladies room had shadowy, rectangular depressions on the wall. Artwork in the ladies room? Upon closer examination, I realized the depressions were urinals, and I was in the men's room.

I raced out the door, past a man standing at a phone kiosk beside the men's room entrance. He stopped talking and gave me a disgusted look. "OK, I made a mistake," I declared. "These things happen."

The experience came to mind after I read Dr. Fran Kaiser's study, "Sexuality in the Elderly." "Until recently, sexual activity in older adults has been considered to be inappropriate, immoral, deviant, or at best, bizarre," she explains. Apparently the man in the phone kiosk thought I was a sexual deviant, voyeur, or pervert.

The truth of the matter is that I am a grandmother on hormone replacement therapy who had a migraine aura that prevented me from reading the sign on the door. Surely I am not the first woman to make this mistake and I probably won't be the last. At least I can laugh about it.

Male Menopause

Of course men don't experience physical menopause, but they do experience some of the psychological symptoms. Doctors are becoming more aware of male menopause and its effects on sexuality. Douglas Schow and his colleagues explain the condition in their study, "Male Menopause: How to Define It, How to Treat It."

The symptoms of male menopause sound a lot like the symptoms of female menopause: hot flashes, depression, sleep problems, lower sex drive, general weakness and lethargy, weight gain, and loss of bone mass. You can imagine the problems that develop when both partners have these symptoms.

Schow and his colleagues think "male menopause will become an increasingly important issue for primary care physicians because the number of men in the United States between the ages of 45–70 years is expected to grow from 46 million in 1990 to 81 million by 2020." They also think more research is needed into the psychological effects of male menopause.

New Definition of Impotence

A new definition of impotence was proposed in a National Institutes of Health Consensus Conference article. The NIH conferences have dual purposes: one, to evaluate existing scientific information, and two, to advance public understanding. Since impotence had become a term with "pejorative implications" the NIH recommended the term "erectile dysfunction."

This is a more accurate term, according to the NIH. Millions of men in our country suffer from erectile dysfunction and the Consensus Conference says:

- Erectile dysfunction increases with age but it isn't inevitable
- Embarrassment keeps patients and health professionals from discussing the problem
- Many cases can be managed with medical therapy
- The diagnosis and treatment of erectile dysfunction must be specific

Erectile dysfunction has a ripple effect, altering partner, family, and work relationships. Raul Schiavi, MD, and Jamil Rehman, MD, detail the causes of erectile dysfunction in their study, "Sexuality and Aging." They say physical health, fear of failure, and relationship with a sexual partner all affect erectile dysfunction. "Marital conflict, problems of commitment and intimacy, power struggles and lack of trust" also contribute to the problem, according to researchers. They point out that men and women tend to blame the man for the cessation of intercourse. Fortunately, many treatments for sexual dysfunction are available.

Treating Male Dysfunction

Before he or she recommends any treatment, a doctor will do a complete physical exam and assess the drugs the patient is taking. Stephen Holzapfel, MD, CCFP, author of "Aging and Sexuality," says drugs can cause sexual dysfunction in men. He includes cardiac, gastrointestinal, neurological, endocrine, oncological, psychiatric, and recreational drugs in his observation.

For example, beta blockers, which are taken to lower blood pressure, may interfere with male erections. Schiavi and Rehman also point out that the erections of aging men may not be as stiff as they used to be. Certainly, sexual dysfunction strikes at the heart of masculinity.

Researchers continue to search for solutions to male dysfunction. Associated Press writer Lauran Neergaard reports on a new medication in her article, "Impotence Pill Gains Approval." In March of 1998 the Food and Drug Administration (FDA) approved Viagra, produced by Pfizer, Inc., to treat impotence. Neergaard notes that Viagra is the first nonsurgical treatment for male impotence that doesn't involve injections or inserting something into the penis. Since Viagra was approved the cost of the pills has risen steadily. The medication is supposed to be used once a day, about an hour before sexual intercourse. Medical experts think Viagra may spur more males into getting help. "Only 5 percent of the estimated 10 million to 20 million impotent Americans get treatment," explains Neergaard, "but the pill could increase that number to 20 percent very quickly."

The public seems to be ignoring the fact that Viagra is not an aphrodisiac and helps dysfunctional men only. An ABC World News Tonight report said demand for the drug has been "enormous." According to ABC, 20,000 prescriptions for Viagra are being filled per day in the United States, and the drug has nearly tripled in price. Viagra has serious side-effects, said ABC, especially when taken with nitrates.

Men who have a low sperm count may benefit from testosterone therapy. This therapy may be oral, intramuscular, or transdermal. As with any therapy, testosterone therapy has some risks, things like weight gain, sleep apnea, and cardiovascular risks.

Douglas Schow and his colleagues cite these and other risks in their study, "Male Menopause: How to Define It, How to Treat It." According to the researchers, aging men usually have decreased serum testosterone levels. However, the researchers think this "plays an insignificant role in the decline of sexual activity."

The question is, should aging men have testosterone replacement therapy? "Testosterone's role in restoring the lost vigor and body composition of youth is questionable," the researchers note. Routine androgen therapy needs to be studied more, say the researchers, and the risks need to be weighed with the benefits.

Impact of Stress on Sexuality

Whether it is unpaid bills, kids on drugs, or added job responsibilities, stress has an impact on sexuality. Phil was a research scientist at a major corporation. His research was so complex that few people understood it, not even his colleagues. Phil's wife had a vague idea of his research, at best. Brilliant, preoccupied, and in his own world, Phil paid scant attention to his appearance, and often had no recollection of driving to the laboratory. Often he worked late into the night. Sexuality became a low priority in Phil's life.

"He is so absorbed in his research that sex doesn't interest him," his wife commented.

When Phil was interested in sex, he was emotionally absent. Although the couple had children, Phil wasn't very involved in their care, or in caring for the couple's sexual relationship. The couple drifted apart until they had parallel lives.

Stress may affect sexuality in unusual ways, ways that require professional help. Contact your doctor if you think stress is affecting your sexuality. Your doctor may refer you to a stress-management program. Get your stress under control as quickly as possible because it can lead to high blood pressure.

Improving Sexuality

Stress management is just one way to improve your sexuality. An essay in the *Mayo Clinic Health Letter* called "Sexuality and Aging" contains some other suggestions. First, older people may have to do some planning before they have intercourse. Long-term estrogen replacement has helped many women. Men have a range of medical options: testosterone medication, vascular surgery, self-injection therapy (injecting medicine into the penis) and new medications. Professional counseling is also an option for both partners. Many couples have improved their sexual relationship by getting away from the daily grind.

Years ago, one of my husband's colleagues told him to attend all of the conferences he could. "My wife and I did that," he said. "Every trip was a honeymoon." Shortly after he made this comment his wife died.

We have followed this advice, traveling when we can, going away for the weekend, or staying home and puttering about the house. Sometimes we just sit on the couch and read. These times are indescribably beautiful. Over the years we have learned to revitalize our sexual relationship in a variety of ways:

- Saying "I love you" every day

- Going out for a romantic dinner

- Enjoying a romantic dinner at home

- Laughing together (my husband cuts out cartoons from the newspaper and gives them to me)

- Surprising each other with small gifts (a hobby magazine, a flowering plant, etc.)

- Leaving love notes around the house

- Giving each other massages

Education seems to be the key to all solutions. You can't benefit from new medical treatments unless you know about them. You can't be helped by an intuitive counselor unless you know what counseling is available. The increasing life span will make sexuality education more important in the years to come.

Sexuality Education

The National Institutes of Health Consensus Development Panel on Impotence has discussed the importance of public education on sexuality. The NIH panel thinks sexual information needs to be distributed via:

- Accurate newspaper and magazine articles
- Radio and television programs
- Special programs at senior citizens centers
- Accurate diagnosis and treatment

Television programs are showing older people in a sexual context, but the portrayals are limited, and some border on ridicule. The print media seems to be doing a better job in the sexuality education department. My hometown newspaper, the *Rochester Post-Bulletin,* published an article, "Courting the 'Golden Years'" by Dawn Schuett.

She cites some U.S. Administration Aging statistics in her article. Life expectancy is 79 years for women and 72 for men. This means "seven out of 10 women born during the 'baby boom' will outlive their husbands," writes Schuett.

In a companion article, "Seniors Put a New Spin on Dating," Schuett says dating is a whole new world for women and men 60 years old and older. These people are young at heart. You would think this would be cause for celebration, but some adult children don't like to see their parents dating. Fixed incomes may put a crimp on dating and women often pay their own way. I think dating in later years shows trust in life. After all, life is for living.

The Need for Touch

From the time we are born until we die, touch is a basic human need. Maya Angelou writes about touch in her book, *Wouldn't Take Nothing for My Journey Now.* In her essay, "Sensual Encouragement," Angelou describes her early days as a dancer. She used makeup to enhance her features and baby oil to make her body shine. Women in the audience would touch Angelou's body when she danced, and call out encouragement to her. At this time of life Angelou realizes the touches were sensual, not sexual, a way for audience members to participate in her dancing.

I think the need for touch increases with age. Touch becomes even more important after an aging person enters a nursing home. Studies show that many nursing home residents, especially those who are demented, may be touch-deprived. Stephen Holzapfel writes about touch in his study, "Aging and Sexuality." "In trying to meet the older person with dementia's need for protection, health care professionals at times forget the equally important need for physical touch and caring," he writes.

Health problems, varicose veins, torn ligaments, muscle spasms, and the like, may change the ways you touch your partner. This doesn't change the need for touch. Talk things over and find other ways to touch your partner.

Cuddling with my husband on a rainy night is one of the most beautiful experiences in life. When my grandchildren hug me I melt. Because I receive touch experiences I know, first-hand, of their emotional benefits. I try to give others the gift of touch, a pat on the hand, a parting hug, and other appropriate gestures.

Ageless Love

The greatest gift we can give someone is the gift of love. Often love is expressed in nonsexual ways. After Mom's doctor told me she would probably die over the weekend I went on "death watch." I had been anticipating my mother's death for months and, suddenly, it was very close, and very real.

At bedtime, I wanted my husband to hold me and listen to my scary thoughts. I wanted the comfort of his arms and his mind. He gave me the comfort I needed. Over and over again, he told me what a wonderful caregiver I had been for Mom.

"You never failed her," he said. "Whatever she needed, you were there." My husband's love buoyed me. With this support I was able to make the final arrangements, write Mom's obituary, and sort through her personal things.

Nevertheless, it was a trying time and I am still working through my grief.

My husband expresses his love with kindness, with touch, and with sexuality. I do the same for him. Yes, we worry about the time when one of us will "go," but we don't dwell on it, and we treat each day as a gift. Romance is alive and well at our house and, apparently, in many other homes.

Los Angeles Times writer Bettijane Levine writes about the eternal spark of romance in her article, "They've Got That Old Feeling: The Giddy Thrill of New Love." She profiles several couples, including Art and Florence Sherman of California, who married in their later years. Art was 78 when they got married and Florence was a sprightly 80. "It's been a wild, passionate roller-coaster ride ever since," Florence is quoted as saying.

Many families of older people are noticing some odd behavior, Levine reports, such as grandparents waiting for the phone to ring, pondering about what to wear on a date, and in some instances, staying out all night. Cell phones are helping the courting process. "Elder love is not very different from any other kind of romantic love," Levine comments.

Love is sexual, intimate, and ageless. The American poet Archibald MacLeish wrote about elder love in his poem, "The Old Gray Couple," included in *The Oxford Book of Aging*. In three verses he paints a word portrait of a couple who "have only to look at each other and laugh." My husband and I have this kind of relationship. These tips will help you to keep the joys of sexuality and intimacy in your life.

Smart Aging Tips

⁓

- Learn more about sexuality in the aging.

- Think of sexuality as a cumulative experience.

- Become aware of the barriers to sexuality, such as health problems, lack of partners, effects of medicine, and Widower's Syndrome.

- Be aware that sexuality is a predictor of general health.

- Stand up for yourself and don't let yourself become sexually invisible.

- Learn about the causes and treatment for sexual dysfunction.

- Discuss the symptoms of menopause and male menopause with your doctor.

- Get professional counseling if stress is interfering with your sexuality.

- Find ways to revitalize your sexual relationship.

- Stay attuned to the medical advances regarding sexuality.

- Give the gift of touch.

- Remember that love is sexual, intimate, and ageless.

6

Making a Difference

We get up with the idea of making a difference in someone's life. But all sorts of transitions—a career change, moving to a new town, kids leaving for college, significant birthdays, death of a loved one, and others—divert our attention. Life's transitions may lead us to an unexpected search for identity.

Two questions loom in our minds:

- Who am I now?
- Where do I go from here?

Before we can make a difference these questions need to be answered. We have to understand our feelings. Feelings have a way of getting jumbled together, and sorting them out can be a slow process. That's the bad news.

The good news: Dr. Richard Carlson and Joseph Bailey, MA, authors of *Slowing Down to the Speed of Life,* say feelings are like a compass. Despite the range, depth, and complexity of our feelings, Carlson and Bailey say they fall into two groups, comfortable and uncomfortable. If we are feeling comfortable we are probably emotionally healthy. On the other hand, if we are feeling uncomfortable we are probably emotionally unhealthy. "They [feelings] let you know which mode of thinking you are in," the authors write.

Feelings lead us to our current definition of happiness, a critical point on the compass. Maturity changes our outlook and the things that used to make us happy may seem trivial now. Poets and philosophers have tried to define happiness for us, but we can only define it for ourselves.

 In order to feel happy I think we have to feel needed, to feel like we are making a difference. My survey respondents had things to say about this subject; here are some quotes:

- "Time to give of yourself."
- "Good feelings for volunteering."
- "More time to enjoy one's children and grand-children."
- "I have no schedule except for my volunteer commitments."
- "Can decide what's most important in life and concentrate on doing those things."
- "Volunteer as much as I am physically able to do (three jobs as of now)."

The widow who wrote the last comment described the life she had made for herself. She watches sunsets and sunrises, enjoys star-gazing, walks around the city, keeps up with magazines and newspapers, and reads one or two books at once. "I have lived today!" she wrote in the margin. Clearly, this is a person who has sustained a zest for life and a strong identity.

Studies show that men and women have vastly different ideas about identity. Marion Zucker Goldstein, MD, and Cathy Ann Perkins, MD, focus on female identity in their study, "Mental Health and the Aging Woman." They say "Women define their identity through relationships of intimacy and care, whereas power and separation secure men's identity."

So when we come to a fork in the road, men and women tend to go in opposite directions. A male retiree may volunteer with the Service Corps of Retired Executives (SCORE). A female retiree may volunteer in a nursing home, or vice versa. Some couples volunteer together to keep a sense of family.

Keep a Sense of Family

The first, and perhaps the foremost, way you can make a difference is by keeping a sense of family. Yesterday, family members used to live in the same area and saw each other frequently. Today, family members are scattered around the globe. With aging comes a deeper appreciation of our family.

In her book, *Soulwork: Clearing the Mind, Opening the Heart, Replenishing the Spirit,* Bettyclare Moffatt writes, "I have learned that families can come together in love, no matter their disparate lifestyles, no matter their unresolved agendas, when a luminous soul draws them together in a circle of unconditional love."

Take steps to keep your family circle together. Send photos, call a loved one, or write a short note. Of course, none of these steps replaces personal contact. Every Sunday our daughter and the twins come for dinner. Old-fashioned as it may sound, this solution works for our family.

In fact, the twins cried once when a blizzard kept them from coming to dinner. Even though they said little when they called us (mostly giggles), the twins were glad to hear our voices. Sunday dinner has become a family tradition, a time to share food, conversation, and love.

Working Together

Some people keep a sense of family by working together. Ann Merrill writes about family members on the job in her article, "Bridging the Generations." The article spotlights Marilyn Carlson Nelson, chief operating officer (COO) of the Carlson Companies, Inc., a Minnesota corporation that generates $4.9 billion dollars in revenue each year and employs about 40,000 people. Curt Carlson founded the travel, marketing, and hospitality corporation some 60 years ago. Marilyn became vice chairman in 1991, and COO in 1997. Her son, Curtis, is president and CEO of Carlson Hospitality Worldwide and her father continues to be involved in the business.

The article says Marilyn has "to decide which of the big rules, the real values this company has been built on, are going to empower us for many generations." One of Marilyn's roles is to act as a go-between with groups, to "try to synthesize the best of the past with the promise of the future."

Family History

You can synthesize the past with the promise of the future by preserving family history. My husband's family came from the Isle of Man, the place where cats have no tails, in the middle of the Irish Sea. According to Manx legend, you can see three kingdoms from the Isle of Man: England, Ireland, and the kingdom of heaven.

My husband and I have been there three times and, although I am not Manx, I felt Manx. With each visit we learned more about the family's history. One relative was imprisoned because he stole a loaf of bread to feed his starving family. I could imagine the ravages of the potato famine, the hunger that made him steal, the scary boat trip to America, and the pioneer spirit that held the family together. I am happy to say this spirit still exists.

Before it's too late, take steps to preserve your family history. Update the family tree, preserve mementos and artifacts, collect and store photos in a safe place, or have a family reunion. Genealogy enthusiasts are using computer programs and the Internet to trace their roots.

Parent Your Adult Children

Being available to our children is another way to make a difference. Parenting adult kids can be a challenge. No parent wants to see their children make poor decisions, yet that is what we must do. It has taken years, but I have finally learned to let go, to allow our daughters to make their own mistakes.

Sure, there have been times when I have winced at their decisions. Couldn't they see the potholes in the road ahead? Apparently not, and no amount of talking would change their minds. All we can do is trust. Adult children will eventually remember the values we instilled in them.

We are available to our daughters and know they will ask for help only if they need it. Our daughters know we will be honest with them. My husband and I are blessed to have come to a time in life when our daughters are our friends. I hope this blessing comes to you.

Grandparenting

You can make a difference by being a grandparent. Until we became grandparents, my husband and I didn't realize how much we needed this role in our lives. We foster contact with our grandchildren because we want to know them. More important, we want them to know us.

Bobb Biehl writes in *Mentoring: Confidence in Finding a Mentor and Becoming One,* "The world in which our children and grandchildren must grow up is far more difficult than the world we experience in our own childhoods." His words make me think of my younger years.

I grew up in trusting times. Mom and Dad didn't lock the doors because nobody would think of walking into our house. Despite a lack of money my childhood was filled with pleasure: catching fireflies, cutting out paper dolls, playing kick the can until dark. Because we didn't have a television set (we got a set when I was a senior in high school) my brother and I became avid readers.

I have tried to give our grandchildren similar pleasures. Each year the twins' school has a special grandparents day. When I peeked through the window of my grandson's room he was doing an alphabet puzzle on the floor. His face lit up when he saw me. My granddaughter threw her arms around me when I walked into her room. I watched the twins play computer games, praised their artwork, and took them to the school book fair. Although I was at school for only an hour, it was a special hour in the twins' lives. We connected. Listening is another way to connect with children.

Listen to Children

It is important for adults to listen to children. Sadly, many children do not have anyone who will listen to them. Make a point to listen to your children, your grandchildren, and the neighborhood kids. Your listening could have long-lasting effects.

One day the twins were drawing chalk pictures on the driveway. I was sitting in a chair watching them. My granddaughter put down the chalk and approached me with an intense look on her face. "Grandma…" she began, fidgeting with her T-shirt. "Grandma…" she said again. Then she took a big breath. "Grandma, my mother would die for me."

Where had this idea come from? My mind raced as I thought of my early childhood training and struggled to frame a reply. I decided my granddaughter wanted reassurance. "Yes," I answered. She smiled, skipped up the driveway, and resumed drawing. The brevity of our conversation does not diminish its importance.

Kids are overprogrammed these days, with dancing lessons, piano lessons, scouts, intramural sports, school plays, club meetings, computer games, and hobbies; they have little time to think. We don't have to fill every moment of their lives. If kids are going to figure things out they need quiet times and, just as important, listening times.

When I hear news stories about teen violence I ask myself, "Is anyone listening?" People of all ages benefit from the gift of listening. Grocery stores, churches, hospitals, and nursing homes are filled with lonely people. You can make a difference in their lives by listening with your ears and your heart.

Grandparents as Parents

Due to drug addiction, alcoholism, running away, and other harmful behaviors, many grandparents are raising their grandchildren. It's not necessarily a welcome role. Lynn Smith writes about the trend in her article, "To Grandmother's House They Go." Observes Smith, "Grandparents want to spoil their grandkids—not raise them."

Exhausted grandparents are joining support groups, such as the California-based "Grandparents As Parents." The American Association of Retired Persons (AARP) runs a clearinghouse for grandparents who are caring for their grandkids, some 400 support groups nationwide.

According to the AARP, approximately 1.5 million kids in our country are being raised by their grandparents. An estimated 2.5 million children are living in their grandparents' home with one parent. Smith thinks life has thrown these people a curve. While they are caring for their grandkids these grandparents are grieving for their adult children. "Many have tried to help their troubled adult children be good parents and are saddened about having to intervene," says Smith.

Some grandparents grapple with their own shortcomings as well. Whether they are toddlers, gradeschoolers, or college age, kids need the support of parents *and* grandparents.

They are confused by their grandparents' dual roles. What do you call the grandparent who is parenting you? One boy, described in Smith's article, calls his grandmother "Nana Mommy."

Raising grandkids is a physical and financial challenge. At a time when grandparents expect to coast, they must find the energy to be parents again. At a time when their home has become an adult place, they must remake it into a safe place for children. That can be hard to do in an older home or apartment.

Associated Press writer Robin Estrin writes about grandparents as parents in " 'Grandfamilies House' Fills a Need," published in the *Rochester Post-Bulletin*. She describes a public housing project in Boston. Funded by private and government funds, the 26 unit complex is the first project designed just for grandparents who are raising grandkids. The grandfamilies house has elevators, ramps, and grab bars for older folks, and safety electrical outlets, window guards, and safe toxic storage for younger folks.

Watch for more information on the grandparents-as-parents issue because the numbers continue to rise. Offer your help to any grandparents in your neighborhood who are raising their grandkids. You may also want to look into building a grandfamilies house in your community.

Be a Caregiver

Caregiving can make a dramatic difference in someone's life. I wrote a book on the subject, *The Alzheimer's Caregiver: Dealing with the Realities of Dementia*, released the week after my mother died. Much as I wanted to talk about my experiences, it was hard to do radio interviews while I was grieving.

Only people who have been caregivers understand what it involves. During nine years of caregiving, I moved my mother three times, monitored her investments, paid her bills, organized her taxes, ran errands for her, made sure she got good medical care, and kept friends apprised of her condition.

Every day I did something for Mom. It has been six

months since she died and I am slowly reclaiming my time. Finding these hours has been like finding gold. I also find comfort in knowing that I did my best. The human lifespan continues to increase and more of us will be caregivers in the years ahead.

Norwegian researcher Eva Skoe and her colleagues report on caregiving attitudes in their study, "The Ethic of Care: Stability Over Time, Gender Differences, and Correlates in Mid-to-Late Adulthood." A total of 60 people, 30 men and 30 women, participated in the first study.

The participants lived in a rural community in eastern Canada and their ages ranged from 60 to 80. Each participant was given an "Ethic of Care Interview," questions about the real-life dilemmas of unplanned pregnancy, marital fidelity, and caring for a parent. All of the participants were interviewed at home.

The researchers found that our approach to caregiving depends on:

- cognitive complexity
- ideas about issues
- opportunities for social interaction
- positive feelings about personal health
- and positive feelings about aging

Women are more apt to focus on the interpersonal aspects of caregiving, according to the researchers, a finding consistent with earlier research. The researchers note that "Caring for others and the self may thus be an aspect of adaptation across the adult life span."

Share Talent and Time

Sharing your talent with others is yet another way to make a difference. Everybody is an expert at something. Barbara, a family friend for decades, was an expert knitter. During her lifetime Barbara knit scores of Fair Isle sweaters, transforming colorful yarn into works of art. She knit so many sweaters the complex pattern was imprinted in her mind forever.

Toward the end of her life, after dementia set in, Barbara could still knit sweaters from memory. She gave most of them away. Like Barbara, we can share our talents with others. We can give them away joyfully, with no strings attached, and no thanks needed.

Even if you aren't a crafter you have something special to share—time. Across the country, from one coast to the other, communities are looking for volunteers. Lisa Berger discusses volunteerism in her book, *Feathering Your Nest: The Retirement Planner,* and says opportunities may be found in such places as:

- churches and temples
- American Red Cross
- Salvation Army
- local museums and libraries
- YMCA and YWCA groups
- Service Corps of Retired Executives (SCORE)

I would add other groups to Berger's list, including:

- American Association of University Women (AAUW)
- service organizations (Lions, Elks, etc.)
- your local history center
- special interest groups, such as quilters
- special community groups (anti-violence groups, ethnic groups)
- Girl Scouts and Boy Scouts

Contact the U.S. government for other volunteer opportunities. A member of the local American Association of University Women, Darlene Vowels, spoke about her work with the Volunteers in Parks (vip) program. Both retired, Darlene and her husband wanted to share their talents with others. After reading an article about vip they sent for information. The Vowels selected the two parks that interested them most and sent off one-page resumes. Darlene and her husband were assigned to the Tonto National Park in Arizona. "It has been one of the top experiences of our lives," Darlene smiled. They have volunteered at Tonto for several years and gained much from the vip program. First, they gained intellectual stimulation; the more the Vowels learned about the Southwest, the more they wanted to know. Volunteering also gave them new opportunities for social interaction.

Physical fitness was a surprising benefit of their volunteerism. The Tonto site requires lots of walking and hiking and the Vowels conducted weekly tours. But the greatest benefit of the vip program was personal satisfaction. "We feel truly needed," Darlene concluded.

Check the *Congressional Quarterly's Washington Information Directory* and the *Encyclopedia of Associations* for more volunteer opportunities. You should be able to find these resources in the reference department of your library.

Do What You Do

To make a difference you don't need to go in a totally new direction. You can keep on doing what you do. In 1994 Minnesota novelist Jon Hassler was diagnosed with Parkinson's disease. A professor at St. John's University in Collegeville for 42 years, he is now emeritus staff.

Elaine Gale updates us on the best-selling author in her article, "The Dean of Writers." Although Parkinson's has slowed him down, he keeps on cranking out prose, and plans to write his memoirs. "There isn't much pain," Hassler is quoted as saying. "I'll get a lot of novels out before it gets me."

The article says Hassler tries to nurture others with his writing. His example—and yours—can make a difference in someone's life. Others may benefit from your talent, training, and the wisdom that comes from experience. Health permitting, you can keep on doing what you do best.

I have noticed that the people who keep on working continue to learn. They keep up with trends, improve their skills, and are usually willing to help others. Getting the job done is an achievement at any age. So is the ability to credit others.

Credit Others

Success doesn't come by itself, it comes from the kindness of others. Give credit where credit is due. Thank your co-workers in person, cite them at meetings, and praise them in print and conversation.

Should you credit those who steered you off course? Yes. They got your creative juices going, made you focus your thinking, and helped you learn from experience. Painful as this learning may have been, you will have acquired valuable life skills.

Compliment others, too. Your compliment doesn't have to be long, but it does have to be genuine. When I received copies of *The Alzheimer's Caregiver* I was so pleased with the care that had gone into the design and layout I called my editor. "It couldn't be better!" I exclaimed. One sentence of praise can warm the heart for years. Turning the spotlight on others takes maturity. It's worth it. Crediting others is a gift for the recipient and the giver.

Link the Generations

Our society has split into layers like a cake, young with the young, old with the old, and baby boomers in the middle. Can we bring these groups together? The Rochester, Minnesota, Public Schools have found a way. Earlene Wickre, coordinator of business services, told me about a program that links adultswith kindergarten students.

The program started in 1997 when 34 adults rode school buses with kindergarten students the first week of school. They helped to enforce safety rules and made sure the kids got off at the right bus stop. Fifty percent of the adults were seniors, and those affiliated with the Senior Citizens Center donated their pay to the center.

"This is one of the best collaborations I've ever seen," Wickre said. "It's great for the kids. It's great for the seniors."

From church guilds, to community action programs, to service groups, you will find many ways to link the generations. We understand each other better when our lives touch. You may touch someone's life by joining a school mentoring program or mentoring on your own.

Be a Mentor

Bobb Biehl discusses the ins and outs of mentoring in his book *Mentoring: Confidence in Finding a Mentor and Becoming One.* Written from a Christian viewpoint, Biehl says mentoring is important because we live in a mobile society.

Minority groups need mentors as well. Kids are struggling with womanhood and manhood and there is an "acute need for healthy models of adult roles and relationships."

In order to be successful mentors Biehl thinks we need to love, encourage, be open, check our motives, and relax. "Anyone can be a mentor," he writes, "but not everyone should." Highly egocentric people and stressed people don't make suitable mentors, according to Biehl.

He tells mentors to set clear boundaries and consider these points before agreeing to a relationship:

1. Time involved

2. Finances (Do you plan to supply materials or loan money?)

3. Needs of the protégé

4. Length of mentorship (one time, one year, ongoing?)

5. Limits of the relationship

6. Any assumptions?

7. Issues that could lead to conflict

8. Are you and your protégé expecting perfection?

9. Special concerns, anxieties

"When it's your time, mentoring is a very significant thing to do," writes Biehl.

Agreeing to be a mentor does not mean you are agreeing to do someone's work for them. In fact, this would deprive your protégé of the satisfaction of rounding the bases, so to speak, of setting goals, working toward them, and achieving them. I don't have the time to join an established mentoring program, but I do have the time to mentor fledgling writers on an informal basis.

A young woman approached me after I spoke at a conference. She asked my opinion about a vague idea for a children's book. This was not the time or the place for an in-depth discussion so I kept my answers brief. Still, the woman kept pestering me with questions.

"What should I write on the first page?" she asked.

"Whatever you want. It's your book."

"I know, but what should the words be?" she persisted. "I can't seem to get started."

I was tempted to say, "It was a dark and stormy night."

It became apparent that the woman didn't want a mentor, she wanted a ghost writer. Since I couldn't write the book for her, I referred her to some writing resources, and told her to make a detailed outline.

"Writing is a slow process," I explained, "a process that requires lots of revisions. You just have to keep at it." The woman left quickly, an angry expression on her face.

My other mentoring experiences have been more satisfying. Helping others makes me feel good, and I've met writers for coffee, had long phone conversations, and typed out notes and recommendations. One grateful writer sent me a beautiful thank-you letter that moved me to tears.

Speak Out

Writers write to make their voices heard. Although you don't need to write books to make your voice heard, you need to speak out in some way, by letter, fax, or E-mail. I wrote a letter to the editor after seeing dozens of people drive through stop signs. You can do the same. The editor, or someone representing the editor, will call to verify your name and address. Keep a copy of your correspondence for future reference.

At social functions you can "stand up and be counted." Don't settle for half truths, distorted truths, or blatant falsehood. You can be the questioning voice or the voice of reason. Short messages are easier to remember than long ones, so be brief, and try not to repeat yourself.

Contact legislators about the issues that concern you.

Lend your name to a cause or get directly involved in community work. There are many ways to make your voice heard. Be courteous because nobody wants to listen to a belligerent person.

Be Courteous

Courtesy still counts. In some parts of the country, however, courtesy is in short supply. Richard Carlson, PhD, points out the advantages of courtesy in his book, *Don't Sweat the Small Stuff ... And It's All Small Stuff.* We should think of strangers as being like ourselves, Carlson says, and treat them with kindness, respect, and eye contact. In the process, "You'll probably notice some pretty nice changes in yourself."

Social customs have changed since my husband and I married. People don't seem to respond to invitations, even if it says RSVP and you have included your phone number. We invited 40 people to a picnic once, and only one couple responded. I had to call people to see if they were coming. It turned out only two people were coming and we canceled the picnic. Since I had already made a variety of breads and salad dressings for the picnic this lack of courtesy was disappointing, to put it mildly. If someone is kind enough to invite us for dinner, I think we should be kind enough to respond.

Business courtesy has also changed since my husband and I married. People I have never seen before call me Hon, Honey, Sweetie, and by my first name. This instant familiarity makes me feel uncomfortable. However, if I know the people these familiar names warm my heart.

Courtesy is a way to show that we care. I try to be courteous to others and leave a smile behind, an approach that didn't work with one business owner. Although she wasn't rude to me, she seemed to be distracted, as if her mind was somewhere else. Each time I was in her shop I tried to get her to smile. One day the woman confided that she had cancer and was undergoing chemotherapy. "I used to plan things and worry about tomorrow," she said. "Now I enjoy today." Our souls connected in that moment and I feel like I have made a friend. As this story illustrates, sometimes courtesy reaps unusual rewards.

Give Money

Charities are competing for our dollars. We can't give money to everyone, but our small check could help a group to reach its financial goal. Telemarketers are calling us day and night, many speaking so fast we can hardly get a word in edgewise. How can we handle these calls?

First, I ask the caller to state the purpose of his or her call in one sentence. As I discovered, few callers can do this. Some callers get flustered by the question because it deviates them from a script.

Second, I ask the caller to send me a brochure or fact sheet. Many callers have no written information to send me.

Third, I don't give out any personal information. My standard reply: "I'm sorry, but we don't answer any phone surveys."

We have whittled our giving down to a few selected groups in self-defense. If you can't donate money, you may be able to donate "time dollars." Just as bartering is a currency of the present, "time dollars" may be the currency of the future. What are they?

Give "Time Dollars"

Kristine Tower explains "time dollars" in her study, "Consumer-Centered Social Work Practice: Restoring Client Self-Determination." Law professor Edgar Cahn came up with the concept, which "involves older people helping others in exchange for future benefits for themselves." The services may include:

- grocery shopping
- cooking meals
- cleaning
- washing, ironing, mending
- driving
- yard work
- patching/painting
- snow shoveling and plowing

- companion services (writing letters, straightening the house, etc.)

At the present time California, Florida, Michigan, Missouri, and Texas have time-dollar programs. Community agencies keep track of the volunteers' time. According to Tower some states guarantee that the volunteer will be able to use his credits even if the program falters.

Thanks to time dollars people have been able to stay in their homes longer. Donors and recipients have more social contacts because of time dollars. And time dollars give volunteers some control over their future needs. If your community doesn't have time dollars you may be able to start a program.

You can make a difference. Giving to others will make your life richer and you will be rewarded a thousand-fold. Instead of feeling defeated, you will have a sense of purpose. As one survey respondent wrote, you will be "aged to perfection."

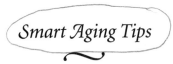

Smart Aging Tips

- Keep a sense of family.
- Be available to your adult children.
- Connect with your grandchildren.
- Listen to children.
- Help out grandparents who are raising their grandkids.
- Become a caregiver and find joy in it.
- Share your time and talents with others.
- Keep on doing what you do.
- Credit others.
- Link the generations.
- Be a mentor.
- Speak out.
- Treat others courteously.
- Donate money or time dollar services.

7

The Joy of Lifelong Learning

No story illustrates the joy of learning like the story of Cyrena Wooster, who earned her high school diploma at the age of 98. As "Good Morning America" co-host Kevin Newman introduced Wooster he said, "You're going to love this story." He was right.

Wooster was there in the studio, sprightly, cheerful, and charming. She told how she quit school in the third grade to care for her 11 siblings. All through her life Wooster longed for a high school diploma. Her reasoning: "So many people have it [their diploma]. I would like to have it too."

With the help of student tutors Wooster earned the diploma she coveted. Math and history were her favorite subjects. "When you're old, it [learning] doesn't come easily," she explained. Wooster credited her tutors for her success. "Every week they came and tutored me … I worked hard, yes."

Newman quickly pointed out that Wooster passed the tests on her own. One tutor was in the studio with Wooster and they held hands during the interview. Clearly, a bond had developed between the two women.

According to the tutor, Wooster's example made other students more appreciative of their diplomas. "It's very inspiring for us all to continue learning," she said. And Wooster, who talked to history students about her life experiences, became a direct connection to living history.

When Wooster pushed her walker across the stage to receive her diploma the students gave her an ovation. Her story was so heartening the television crew burst into spontaneous applause at the end of the interview. Cyrena Wooster proved the human mind can continue to learn.

Is she an exception? Researchers are studying how the mind stores and retrieves data. Studies show that exercising the mind helps to keep it active. The saying, "Use it or lose it" may be applied to learning. We must figure out how to use our minds as we age.

Studies on Learning

One study, "The Influence of Summary Knowledge of Results and Aging on Motor Learning," by Heather Carnahan and her colleagues, compares undergraduate students with senior citizens. The study's purpose was "to examine whether adults use summary KR [knowledge of results] to facilitate learning in a manner similar to young adults."

You might bet on the students because their minds absorb information like sponges. But this experiment had some startling results.

Twenty-four students and 24 senior citizens participated in the study. What makes the study interesting is its method. The experiment had two phases, acquisition and retention. First, the participants were asked to learn a sequence on a computer keypad within a specified length of time. Then, using the index finger of their dominant hand, they were asked to repeat the sequence within 1200 milliseconds.

Both students and seniors did better when they received a knowledge of results (KR), commonly called feedback, after every trial, as opposed to every five trials. "The positive finding in regard to aging is that older subjects were able to benefit during retention from summary KR lengths of five trials in a manner similar to young adults."

Carnahan and her colleagues think more research on complex tasks is needed. Encouraging as their research may be, lapses in memory occur, and we sometimes talk around a subject or stop talking altogether. Our minds cannot retrieve data on command. A friend calls these times "senior moments" and I like her term.

Delayed Recall

Senior moments are actually delayed recall. Warren Gorman, MD, and Chris Campbell, JD, discuss delayed recall in their study, "Mental Acuity of the Normal Elderly." They explain that aging people may forget facts, things like names and dates and events "when these events are not critical in their lives." I understand this.

My mind is packed with information and I figure there is only so much space left for new stuff. So I don't try to remember everything. Besides, I can always look up information later if I need it. Computer databases have made research easier, faster, and fun.

Anyone who has experienced delayed recall knows how frustrating it can be. Senior moments may be embarrassing for the speaker and the listener. However, the researchers say delayed recall isn't constant or debilitating. It may take minutes, hours, or days, but the facts we are seeking usually come to mind.

Cued Recall

Dr. David Friedman and his colleagues examine memory in their study, "Implicit Retrieval Processes in Cued Recall: Implications for Aging Effects in Memory." They conducted an experiment to test the mind's retrieval system. The purpose of the experiment was to study indirect memory and direct memory. Indirect memory is used to "process a stimulus on line without explicit mention of a prior episode." Whereas direct memory is used "to think back to a prior episode."

Forty younger subjects, with a mean age of 26.4 and 40 older subjects, with a mean age of 69.8, joined in the experiment. Younger subjects had more education than the older. All of the older subjects were dementia- and depression-free. The experiment had several phases. During the study phase the participants were exposed to two groups of words, alphabetical and animal. During the testing phase words were flashed on a computer screen. The participants were asked to identify words they had seen before (direct memory) and to complete some words (indirect memory). What happened?

"Contrary to previous research, older subjects produced equivalent performance to young subjects on the direct test as well as the indirect test," they write. Dr. Friedman and his colleagues suspect the test's difficulty influenced the results. Still, the results give us food for thought.

Estrogen Therapy and Dementia

Some experts think estrogen therapy keeps the mind alert. Stanley Birge, MD, titles his study, "Is There a Role for Estrogen Replacement Therapy in the Prevention and Treatment of Dementia?" Estrogen deficiency in postmenopausal women may contribute to the mental changes associated with dementia, according to Birge.

Studies suggest that estrogen has an effect on the brain's neurons. This being the case, will estrogen replacement cure dementia? It depends on the cause.

Birge says there is increasing medical evidence that estrogen replacement "may not only prevent the development of vascular disease but also improve blood flow in women with existing vascular disease." He cites small, nonrandomized studies of estrogen replacement therapy. Improvement was significant in depressed patients over 70 who had mild Alzheimer's disease. "Because the improvement in cognitive function in most of the subjects was associated with an improvement in depressive symptoms, it is difficult to conclude that the changes in cognitive function are attributed to a direct and independent effect of estrogen on this domain of mental function."

The estrogen issue continues to be debated. Birge thinks replacement therapy should be used with caution in menopausal women and sees a need for more clinical trials.

I've been on estrogen so long, I feel like a one-woman clinical trial. For me, the decision to stop taking estrogen is a scary one. Will my IQ drop like a stone? Will I be less creative? Will I shrink another inch? Other women share my concerns.

When the time comes, I will make the decision based on medical research and my doctor's advice. But I'm not ready to give up on estrogen yet. Hormone replacement therapy (HRT) has been good to me. I am more creative now than I have ever been and, while I can't prove it, this may be due to estrogen.

An article in the Alzheimer's Association newsletter, "Studies Provide Further Insight Into Alzheimer's," talks about estrogen therapy. It says recent studies have shown that hormone replacement therapy "may have a protective effect on nerve cells in the brain." Researchers aren't sure how estrogen works, but know it is "involved in nerve cell protection."

Importance of Early Education

Education may help to prevent mental aging, according to Warren Gorman, MD, and Chris Campbell, JD, authors of "Mental Acuity of the Normal Elderly." Studies show aging people with a higher education do better than aging people with less education on mental tests. The researchers note, "An increased amount of early formal education may delay, or perhaps even prevent, the dulling of mental acuity which takes place with normal aging."

This finding should make us feel good about the education we have and, more important, whet our intellectual curiosity. I took French in high school and, although I wasn't a stellar student, I enjoyed the language. Several years ago, possibly due to aging, French words started to wake me up at night.

They were odd words, such as *oeuf,* which means egg. So many words percolated into my consciousness I decided to take French lessons. I took lessons until the demands of caregiving took over my life. Despite a poor accent, I enjoyed the musical language and learning to think in French. The most valuable lesson: I could still learn.

Teaching Methods

New teaching methods are being developed for the aging. Sally Weinrich, PhD, RN, and her colleagues describe some of these methods in their study, "Teaching Older Adults by Adapting for Age Changes." According to the researchers, few cancer education programs have been tailored to meet the needs of the elderly.

The American Cancer Society recommends fecal occult blood screening (FOBS) yearly after the age of 50. Weinrich and her colleagues developed a visual program to show how the screening works. Used at eight randomly selected meal sites for the elderly in the South, the program:

- allowed more time for learning
- included posters about FOBS testing
- included pictures that showed the procedure
- used peanut butter to demonstrate the procedure

- gave participants reminder notes on when to return their kits
- adapted written materials to a fifth grade reading level

You may laugh about the peanut butter (I did) but it served its purpose. "Teaching the elderly varies more in how we teach than in what we teach," the researchers write. Visual teaching methods may be adapted to other situations. The point of this story is to know the people you are teaching.

Overlearning

Warren Gorman, MD, and Cris Campbell, JD, write about a proven memory system in their study, "Mental Acuity of the Normal Elderly." For years actors and speakers have used visual clues to remember information. As the researchers explain, "The subject associates the item to be overlearned with a visual image that already is a familiar one."

Overlearning works even when you're stressed. I wrote a book on the history of Rochester, Minnesota, and was asked to talk about it to a community group. Being a planner, I put my book and speech outline on the podium, and waited to be introduced. When I reached the podium the outline was gone and I could hardly believe my eyes. This was a speaker's worst nightmare. Hours of work had gone into the outline and I wondered if I would remember it. "Are my notes in my briefcase?" I asked a friend in the audience.

"I don't see them," she answered with a weak smile.

Thank goodness fate was with me. In addition to being the author of the book, I was also the photo researcher. I had found historic photos, had special photos taken, and written all of the captions. Not only did I remember the photos, I remembered their chapter locations.

These visual clues enabled me to give a cogent talk. Try overlearning if you need to remember information. Some people think of humorous visuals to make them more memorable. "It is never too late to practice learning to remember," say Gorman and Campbell.

Teaching Materials

New materials are being developed to teach the aging. Ireta Ekstrom, MEd, details some of these materials in her study, "Printed Materials for an Aging Population: Design Considerations." According to Ekstrom, roughly 85 percent of learning occurs through vision.

Physical changes, such as fatigue, chronic pain, hearing loss, and poor vision, may hinder learning. Ekstrom writes, "Many learning difficulties stem from deficiencies in vision since our vision becomes less acute with aging." Even if we wear glasses we may have trouble reading.

Most printed materials can be improved in one way or another. Ekstrom says printed materials need to be readable. Readability is determined by type, spacing, and word and line length. Printed materials also need to be legible. Legibility is determined by the speed of word recognition, a complex decoding process.

Ekstrom says we should avoid:

- printing letters on a patterned background
- glossy paper (too shiny)
- metallic inks (too much glare)
- reverse type (light letters on a dark background)
- overly large or overly small type
- enlarging smaller print with a copy machine (results may be fuzzy)
- printing words in capital letters

Printed materials should be crisp and clear. Type with a serif is usually easier to read. Line lengths should be 50 to 70 characters per line, with clear headings, extra spacing, and unjustified margins. "Older adults will require certain kinds of considerations because of the more pronounced influence of aging, but younger adults are also aging, even though they may not need as many adjustments to accommodate to learning," notes Ekstrom.

To my knowledge, no comprehensive study of printed materials for the aging has been conducted. However, I suspect that Ekstrom's recommendations would make learning easier for all of us. Eye-catching colors and graphics make printed materials more appealing.

Size is important too. Toward the end of his life, when my father was in the firemen's home, I sent him a book about fire engines. A one-volume encyclopedia, the book was packed with photos, and I thought it would give him hours of pleasure. Things didn't work out that way.

"It's a nice book, Harriet," he said. "But it's so heavy I can hardly hold it." We need to keep size and weight in mind when designing printed materials for the aging. Paperback books weigh less than hardcover and slip easily into a purse, briefcase, or backpack.

Smoking and Mental Ability

Smoking is becoming less attractive in our society.

Dr. Daniel Galanis and his colleagues examine the association between smoking history and mental ability in their study, "Smoking History in Middle Age and Subsequent Cognitive Performance in Elderly Japanese-American Men." The question: Could smoking contribute to vascular dementia and mental impairment?

A total of 3,429 Japanese-American men, who were part of the Honolulu Heart Program and the Honolulu Aging Study, participated in the study. All of the participants were given mental ability tests. They were also asked to classify themselves as "never," "former," or "current" smokers. The well-documented smoking histories are a major strength of the study, according to the researchers.

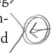The data indicated that smoking may contribute not just to vascular dementia, but to Alzheimer's disease, a finding that conflicts with earlier research. "We conclude that continuous smoking in middle age is associated with increased cognitive impairment later in life among these men."

The study made me think of the latest research on passive smoke. Apparently passive smoke is more dangerous to other people in the room than to the smoker. I lived in a smoke-filled environment—my home—for 19 years. My mother lived in it for decades. Did my father's smoking contribute to her dementia?

Smoking and Alzheimer's

The British medical journal, *The Lancet,* contains a study about smoking titled "Smoking and Risk of Dementia and Alzheimer's Disease in a Population-Based Cohort Study: The Rotterdam Study." It is the first prospective study of smoking ever conducted.

A. Ott, PhD, and other colleagues studied 6,870 dementia-free older people in Rotterdam. Detailed smoking histories were taken. The participants were divided into three groups for study purposes: never smokers, former smokers, and current smokers.

In two years, 146 of the participants had dementia and 105 had Alzheimer's. Smokers had a higher risk for Alzheimer's, actually 2.3 times the risk, than nonsmokers. And smokers who had the Alzheimer's gene were four times more likely to get the disease.

The evidence against tobacco is mountainous. Heart disease. Lung disease. Hearing loss. Mouth cancer. Gray skin. Stained fingers. Possible dementia. Be kind to yourself. If

you are a smoker, enroll in a smoking cessation program,
and do your best to stop.

Driver Improvement Courses

We've seen how smoking may damage our minds. What about the minds of older drivers? Driving safety is a thorny issue in an aging population. The number of older drivers is soaring, according to Nikiforos Stamatidis and John Deacon, authors of "Trends in Highway Safety: Effects of an Aging Population on Aging Propensity."

Between 1970 and 1990, the number of older drivers increased 170 percent. Female drivers increased a startling 270 percent during this time.

Americans don't just love their cars, we are dependent on them. "Dependence of the elderly on the personal automobile has been intensified by increased suburbanization and deteriorating public transportation services," say the researchers.

Using historical accident data, driver's age, cohort, gender, year of accident, location, and lighting, the researchers determined accident propensity. Some of the results:

- Middle-aged drivers are safer than younger drivers.

- Younger drivers are generally safer than older drivers.

- Female drivers are safer on average than male drivers.

- Younger female drivers are safer than older female drivers.

- Older male drivers are safer than older female drivers.

The researchers consider older drivers "a high-risk component of the future driving population." That's why insurance companies are offering discounts to seniors who take driver improvement courses. Reviewing the rules of the road is helpful to all drivers. The American Automobile Association (AAA) publishes a helpful brochure, "The Older and Wiser Driver." Call your local office to get a copy. Ask about the AAA national driver improvement program for senior citizens. Check with your local AAA office because not all states have the program. The initial course lasts eight hours and covers:

- communicating in traffic situations
- keeping a margin of safety
- driving emergencies
- vehicle maintenance
- making responsible decisions about alcohol, fatigue, and feelings

Course participants get helpful brochures, see videos, and receive an attendance certificate for insurance purposes. For example, USAA in San Antonio, Texas, gives policy holders a 10 percent discount on their car insurance if they have taken a driver improvement course.

Your local senior citizens center may have a similar driver improvement program. Maybe more of us need a driver improvement course because aggressive driving is increasing in our nation.

Richard Carlson, PhD, in his book *Don't Sweat the Small Stuff... And It's All Small Stuff,* urges us to be less aggressive drivers. He has good reasons for this advice. Aggressive driving puts us and other drivers in danger. Dealing with aggressive drivers is a stressful experience.

Experts say aggressive driving tactics—following too close, weaving in traffic, and speeding—save little time. I was writing a newspaper article about the "55 Alive" course at the senior citizens center and sat in on one of the sessions. The instructor said speeding saves, on average, only two minutes.

Let the aggressive drivers pass you. Chances are, you will meet them at the next red light.

Elderhostel

An increasing number of older people are giving Elderhostel the green light. Elderhostel is a nonprofit group "committed to being the preeminent provider of high quality, affordable, educational opportunities for older adults," according to its quarterly catalogs. You must be 55 years old or older to participate in the programs. Spouses and companions are also eligible.

Catalogs are published in spring, summer, winter, and fall. To get a catalog write Elderhostel, 75 Federal Street, Boston, Massachusetts 02112-1941. You may also call 617-426-7788 for information. Elderhostel publishes a Canadian catalog, an international catalog, various supplements, and a special catalog of service programs.

Elderhostel also has an academic program. There is no homework, except for Intensive Studies, and no tests or grades are given. The academic program fee covers:

- accommodations ("plain and simple" according to the catalogs)
- meals (no special diets, please)
- extracurricular activities

Your travel fees are not covered. However, the catalogs list the types of transportation that are available: bus, plane, train, ferry, or stay-over. Trips and courses are listed in the catalogs alphabetically by state. I was curious about Minnesota so I looked up the state listings and they included: a language camp; Mayo Clinic seminars, including "What's New In Health Care"; and Lake Superior history, geology, biology, and beauty.

Service trips are detailed in a video, "Elderhostel Service Programs: Adventures That Make a Difference." The 14-

minute action video costs $6.00. To order the video write to Service Video, in care of the address listed above.

American Association of University Women
The American Association of University Women (AAUW) fosters lifelong learning for women. You must have a four-year college degree in order to join. Members may participate in book clubs, study groups, and social groups. Each AAUW branch raises funds for student scholarships.

When you join the AAUW you receive its national magazine, state newspaper, and local newsletter. You may also attend national and state conventions. Special resources and merchandise, including a membership directory, are available.

Call 800-326-2289 to learn more about the AAUW. You may also fax the AAUW at 202-872-1425. Or write to 1111 16th Street NW, Washington, DC 20036-4873. Your best source of information is an AAUW member. Visit a meeting to see the group in action.

Study/Book Clubs
Study clubs are ideal places to learn. During the course of its history Rochester, Minnesota, has had a variety of study clubs for women. They had similar names and most of them met on Mondays. An outgrowth of the Chautauqua movement, the study clubs gave women the equivalent of a high school education. I belong to a club that was founded in 1892.

Each year we vote on a study topic and we have studied many interesting things: countries, races, history, authors, agriculture, islands, and more. "Potpourri" is a favorite topic because it gives members a chance to read about their personal interests. This year I am giving a paper on buttons.

"You can't talk for an hour about buttons," a member declared.

"I can talk for two hours about buttons!" I retorted.

I consider buttons miniature works of art. Because of Study Club I purchased a beautiful art book, joined the National Button Society, learned about the button blankets used by northwest coast Indian groups, and perused buttons at area stores. I became more aware of buttons in general.

You may think I have lost my mental buttons. I haven't. Belonging to the study club has broadened my friendships and my mind.

Joining a book club is another way to keep your mind active. AAUW has a variety of book clubs, as do many churches. Bookstores are starting clubs to generate customer interest. Usually book club members receive a discount on their purchases. Check your newspaper for book club notices, author appearances, and free talks.

Distance Education

Colleges and universities are offering innovative study programs. The University of Minnesota has a Distance Education program, courses given over the computer network. Debbie Hillengass, the program director of Distance Education, said the program links students all over the world.

"We have students in Russia and the South Pole," she explained. The University of Minnesota offers courses in 80 different academic departments and they cover the alphabet—everything from accounting to women's studies. Students may register in person, by mail, by fax, or by computer. Homework is sent in by electronic mail or the US mail.

The University of Minnesota is offering more courses in a term-based format. "People who are living in a senior residence could register individually and meet in a group," Hillengass said. Students can earn a Bachelor of Applied Business degree through Distance Education.

The Compleat & Practical Scholar is another innovative program at the University of Minnesota. Program Director Susan Lindoo said courses under the Compleat Scholar program are mostly in the liberal arts. Courses under the Practical Scholar program focus on personal interests, such as gardening.

"The program size always fluctuates some," said Lindoo. In past years the university has received 4,000 to 5,000 registrations. Students in the Compleat & Practical Scholar programs attend courses on-campus or at community sites.

Graduate students may tailor a Master of Liberal Arts degree to meet their interests and needs. It is "rigorous and relevant" study, according to the program brochure. Students learn disciplinary approaches to learning, understand "the importance and the difficulty of inquiry," learn about current research and "cutting-edge technology," and study topics that are important to them.

Call the university or college nearest you and ask about their new study programs. There are many learning opportunities out there and we may as well take advantage of them.

Learning from Experience

We may also learn from life experience. If you were to stick a microphone in my face and ask me what life had taught me, I would give you a concise list.

LIFE IS LOVING. There is no limit to love and it continues to grow. Since love cannot be measured there is no point in trying to measure it. We can savor love and the beauty it brings to ordinary days.

LIFE IS CARING AND SHARING. No matter where we live or what we do, we all have similar needs. Caring about others makes us feel good and helps others.

LIFE IS KEEPING AT IT. I wouldn't be a writer without persistence: doing the research, typing the manuscript, keeping up with publishing, and coming up with new book ideas. I am glad persistence is part of my personality.

LIFE IS PAIN. Although we cannot escape the pain of life, we can grow from it. Painful times give us insights we would not have had otherwise. If I had not been grieving for my mother I would probably not have written two books about Alzheimer's disease.

LIFE IS SHORT. That we are alive is amazing and I don't take it for granted. My father-in-law snaps his fingers to demonstrate the shortness of his life. I think life is too short for grudges and, while we might not forget, we can find the courage to forgive.

LIFE IS NOW. I have learned to appreciate the moment.

Richard Carlson and Joseph Bailey talk about immediacy in their book, *Slowing Down to the Speed of Life*. They write, "Living in the moment helps us slow down from our crazy pace and live our lives guided by wisdom."

Wisdom

What is wisdom? I think it is the combination of intelligence, integrity, and experience. As we grow older we have many chances to share the wisdom of our experience with others. We have to do this carefully, however, and not force our way into people's lives.

Younger people often trade enthusiasm for experience. Although this may lead to positive outcomes, it ignores the talents and experiences of others. Lacking this input, less experienced people may spend valuable time reinventing old stuff. "If only they would listen a little bit," a grandmother sighed. "We could help them so much."

You must decide when to share the wisdom of your experience. Minneapolis *Star Tribune* writer Kristin Tillotson discusses wisdom in her article, "When We Appraise Our Assets, Gray Matters." She tells readers to call the elderly neighbor next door if they need help. "Wrinkles don't rub off," says Tillotson, "but wisdom can."

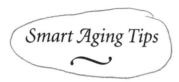

Smart Aging Tips

- Keep the joy of learning in your life.
- Use feedback to help you learn.
- Remember that delayed recall isn't critical and isn't debilitating.
- Ask your doctor about the effects of estrogens on mental ability.
- Use visual cues (posters, demonstrations, overlearning) to help you remember.
- Choose magazines, newspapers, and other printed materials that are readable and legible.

- Stop smoking, if you are still doing it, and avoid passive smoke.
- Take a driver improvement course.
- Go on an Elderhostel trip.
- Join a study or book club.
- Investigate distance education and other learning programs.
- Learn from experience.
- Share your wisdom with others.

8

Mapping Your Future

Start to map your future now. While having a map won't guarantee how your life will go, it will make you think ahead. You need to be aware of recent trends in order to make a map. Three of the trends are: saving less, new retirement procedures, and "economic outpatient care," a term for financially dependent kids.

Saving Less

Saving money for a rainy day isn't a popular idea, according to David Wise, author of the study, "Retirement Against the Demographic Trend: More Older People Living Longer, Working Less, and Saving Less." The Harvard economist says financial experts worry about the low savings rate in America because it may limit future economic growth.

Wise thinks the decline in the labor force corresponds to the start of the Social Security program. Despite corrective measures, many economists predict Social Security will run out of funds. To complicate matters more, about half of American workers are covered by employer pension plans, some three-quarters of which are determined by a formula.

What happens if the formula isn't in your favor? You may decide to quit earlier or work longer. However, working longer may not increase your retirement benefits. Before you make a hasty decision, check your retirement plan carefully. Meet with retirement counselors and get their advice.

Baby boomers are being financially assaulted from several directions. College costs are escalating. Many boomers, who waited to have their children, are paying for college while they are also supporting their failing parents. College-bound kids may choose an exclusive school instead of a state school, which kites costs.

How much should you save for college and retirement? I can't tell you. However, you can get more information by writing the American Savings Education Council, 2121 K Street NW, Suite 600, Washington, DC 20037-1896. The council has a work sheet on the Internet at http://www.asec.org.

You may operate on the theory that saving something is better than saving nothing. This is partly true. But journalist Hank Ezell says in his article, "Retirement Planning: Most of Us Way Behind," many workers have saved only "meager sums." These savings may not be enough for the years ahead. Your retirement income will probably be less than your employed income. And the road to retirement is not the straight, out-to-pasture road it used to be. Retirement policies and procedures have changed a lot.

Changes in the Retirement Process

Glen Elder, Jr., and Eliza Pavalko discuss retirement changes in their study, "Work Careers in Men's Later Years: Transitions, Trajectories, and Historical Change." Men don't always suddenly stop working, but they may have a partial retirement, work at "bridge jobs" (a job between the end of their career and full retirement), or find other work after retirement.

Elder and Pavalko identify five possible retirement patterns in their longitudinal study:

1. Gradual reduction in the time worked

2. Significant reduction in the time worked

3. Exit from the workforce

4. Abrupt exit from the workforce (workers may be victims of down-sizing, corporate restructuring, buyouts)

5. No transition time (due to death and other causes)

Interestingly, men who were in poor health in their 50s were not likely to retire early. Being self-employed didn't decrease the chances of abrupt retirement.

"Work in later life represents a dynamic process that may involve movement into entirely new forms of work as well as reductions in the time worked," the researchers say.

You need to start thinking about retirement well before your retirement date. My father started receiving brochures two years before he was slated to retire. If I remember correctly, one brochure was titled, "Do You Know You're Going to Retire?"

The title made Dad angry when he saw it. He read the title aloud and added sarcastically, "No kidding!" Although we may not like the titles, brochures and booklets about retirement are helpful. You might want to start a file of information.

Retirement Date

The date of your retirement depends on a variety of factors. Mary Anne Taylor and Lynn McFarlane Shore detail some of these factors in their study, "Predictors of Planned Retirement Age: An Application of Beehr's Model." Using a 1986 model of retirement, the researchers studied 264 people employed in a large firm in the southeastern part of the country. The participants (mostly men) completed two surveys.

One major finding of the study: age, health, and finances are major predictors of retirement. Employees with nondebilitating health problems may work to receive their medical benefits. Other employees may work longer to hedge against inflation.

You have probably met people who are afraid to retire. Their reasoning goes something like this: "Fred (or some other name) retired early and was dead within six months. I'm not going to retire!" These people, and you may be one of them, link retirement with death.

Job satisfaction plays a part in your retirement date. To cut costs, many businesses have established hiring freezes and are asking their existing employees to work harder. The fact of the matter is humans can only work so hard. Why kill yourself?

Some workers are threatened by technological advances, such as computer networks. Instead of learning new skills they choose to retire. Often these people have specific goals for retirement, such as visiting grandchildren, touring the country, and pursuing new interests.

"Those who are prepared for retirement may view it more positively," note the researchers. Other factors may also determine your retirement date. For example, you may want to see a project through to completion.

Work Sites and Situations

Geriatric researcher Sara Czaja tells about changing employment in her study, "Employment Opportunities for Older Adults: Engineering Design and Research Issues." According to Czaja, "As the percentage of older workers with full-time jobs has decreased, the percentage of part-time workers has increased with age." Low wages are forcing many older workers to retire earlier than anticipated. This is a terrible waste of talent.

Aging is one of the reasons I became a writer. I choose my own projects, set my own hours, and work at home. Writing enables me to be in two worlds at once, business and home, and I love them both. While I am writing, soup is simmering on the stove, bread is baking in the oven, and the laundry equipment is churning away.

Although I have a computer, I keep a pencil and pad in my purse so I can write anywhere. I will write as long as my brain works. Contacts in the publishing industry treat me kindly, courteously, and respectfully. I am blessed.

Many employers treat older workers poorly; society will eventually pay for this. As Czaja writes, "Unless strategies are developed to either retain older people in the workforce or have them reenter after retirement from their primary occupation, the issues of economic dependency are likely to become formidable in the near future."

Are there any solutions in sight? Czaja, who is in the Department of Industrial Engineering at the University of Miami, thinks employers have options:

- Training programs for older workers (computer, use of new equipment, etc.)

- Redesigning the workplace (traffic patterns, noise abatement, privacy, etc.)

- Redesigning jobs (which may involve combining two smaller jobs into one)

- Changing equipment design

- Interventions "that would offset declines in performance"

Research has shown that older people can be retrained successfully, Czaja says, if the right training methods are used. Some older workers don't need training and continue to work. Younger workers may look to older workers for guidance.

Financially Dependent Kids

The best financial plans may go astray. An increasing number of parents have children in their mid-30s and early 40s who are financially dependent on them. One reason we pay for our children's college education is to make them financially independent. How long do we have to support our children?

Thomas Stanley, PhD, and William Danko, PhD, authors of *The Millionaire Next Door,* think the constant giving to adult children is a mistake. Some parents feel compelled, and even obligated, to give money to adult children and their families. The result is economic outpatient care, or EOM.

It is no surprise that parents with children on economic outpatient care have less money for themselves. Economic outpatient care in America is widespread, according to the authors. Giving money to adult kids may not necessarily be helpful. "In general, the more dollars adult children receive, the fewer they accumulate, while those who are given fewer dollars accumulate more," they write.

Stanley and Danko also say adult children who are waiting for the next check "are not very productive." While they are not in favor of economic outpatient care, they make an exception for daughters. Female workers tend to be paid less than male so parents are more willing to share their money with them.

Giving money to children when they are well into adulthood may undermine their self-respect. Adults want to be independent, and being on the dole keeps them in a dependent relationship. I don't want this for my children or myself.

Financial Planning

Financial planning isn't a weekend project. It can take months. How ever long it takes, financial planning should be a point on your life map. Where do you start? Lisa Berger, author of *Feathering Your Nest: The Retirement Planner,* has a five-step planning process.

STEP 1: Calculate your net worth. This includes savings, real estate, cars, stocks, bonds, insurance policies, savings funds, antiques, etc. Berger says your net worth is a snapshot of the retirement date you have selected. Your snapshot may change as your life changes.

STEP 2: Calculate your sources of retirement income. Will your pension be significantly lower than your salary? Will you receive stock dividends? What is your Social Security stipend? Are you entitled to any other funds?

STEP 3: Add up your current assets. How much would you get if you sold your assets on your retirement date? Don't put a high value on personal property, cautions Berger, because you will probably not want to part with these things.

STEP 4: Add up all of your liabilities. How much do you owe on your mortgage? Do you have a large credit card balance? Are you paying alimony? Do you have any outstanding medical bills?

STEP 5: Figure the difference between step four and step five. Berger says "a small, or even negative, net worth is cause for concern but not panic, unless you plan to retire soon." A large negative balance is cause for concern.

Berger has a mathematical formula for determining your financial needs in retirement. The formula is based on income, expenses, years to retirement, estimated rate of inflation, and annual expenses. You must decide if you want to maintain a similar lifestyle or live less expensively.

Starting a College Fund

One goal of your financial plan may be a college fund for children or grandchildren. *New York Times* columnist Pamela Kruger examines costs in her article, "Baby Boomers Find Themselves Unprepared for the High Cost of College." She thinks parents are getting smarter. Young couples are setting up college funds for their kids, and in some instances, before the kids are born.

Setting up a college fund can be tricky business. You cannot be sure of the inflation rate, for one thing. Economic blips on the other side of the world may affect our economy for years. Jeff Brown tells about some of the complications in his article, "College-Age Kids, Retirement Budget." He cautions parents about putting funds in a student's name because these funds may not be used for four years of college. Trust funds should not be put in a student's name "even if they don't have access to the money until after their college years." Students may be eligible for financial aid.

There are many factors to consider in establishing a college fund. Some parents put stocks and/or dividends in an unmarked fund for college use. It's a good idea to consult a financial advisor. When it comes to college funds, Jeff Brown says planning is the key.

Legal Planning

Legal planning should be another point on your map. If you haven't taken the time to make a will, do it now. This is one way to protect your loved ones. Laws change and even if you have a will, it might be a good idea for a lawyer to review it.

Review your will every five years. Gather your legal documents together and put them in a safe deposit box. You should have:

- Two copies of your will
- Birth certificates
- Marriage certificate
- Power of attorney documents
- Living will documents, if you have decided to do that
- Cemetery and burial documents
- Trust documents
- Insurance policies

You may want to photocopy some of these documents. Insurance companies change, too, so check on current addresses and phone numbers. You might also want to think about making a living will.

Five Wishes Living Will

James Towey, president of the Commission on Aging With Dignity, reported on a new kind of living will on the *Today* television show. He is the founder of the Five Wishes Living Will which covers:

1. Medical care

2. Comfort level

3. Attitudes on caregivers

4. What loved ones should know

5. Who should make decisions

"The right to be treated with dignity is an inherent right," Towey said on *Today*. The Five Wishes Living Will is written in simple English and no attorney is needed. Towey's appearance on the *Today* show generated 100,000 requests in less than two months. I wrote for information about the will and in a September 1997 letter Towey said: "Five Wishes gives you the opportunity to make all of your wishes known, and have your God-given dignity known."

Originally written for Florida residents, Towey noted that the will may have to be adapted for your state. To learn more about the Five Wishes Living Will write to PO Box 1180, Tallahassee, Florida 32302-3180. You may also call 800-681-2010 or fax 850-681-2481.

Long-Term Care Insurance

More Americans are buying long-term care insurance. Why? They want the security of knowing they have medical care in their later years. "A Shopper's Guide to Long-Term

Care Insurance," published by the National Association of Insurance Commissioners, explains that long-term care is many services. The services are "aimed at helping people with chronic conditions." Although you cannot predict the need for long-term care, you can plan for it.

Despite changing statistics, women still outlive men, so more women will need long-term care in their later years. "The chances of needing home health care are substantially greater than needing nursing home care," according to the National Association of Insurance Commissioners.

Your life insurance company may sell long-term care policies. Or you may be able to buy a policy from your employer, from an association, or from a state partnership. Read the benefits section carefully. Be aware of which services are covered and which are not.

Also be aware of what may trigger these benefits:

- Inability to perform the activities of daily living
- Mental impairments (dementia, Alzheimer's disease)
- Physician's orders
- In some instances, prior hospitalization

Ask the insurance agent if you can buy inflation protection. If you don't have this feature, you may own a policy that doesn't cover your medical expenses. The National Association of Insurance Commissioners says a nursing home that costs $86 a day now will cost $220 in only 20 years.

The Association offers these tips for buying long-term care insurance.

1. Ask lots of questions.

2. Shop around; check with several companies.

3. Take your time.

4. Read the policy and make sure you understand it.

5. Don't let advertising and hard-sell tactics sway you.

6. Buy one policy only. (Shooting money in a variety of directions may not help you.)

7. Disclose your medical history.

8. Pay by check, not cash, so you have a receipt.

9. Write down the agent's name, address, phone number, toll-free number, fax number, and E-mail address.

10. Contact the agent if you don't receive the policy within 60 days.

11. Review the policy again during the "free-look period."

12. Read the insurance application again.

13. Consider having the premiums automatically paid by your bank account.

Do not answer any questions over the phone about Medicare or your current insurance, the commissioners caution. They also say we should be wary of letters and cards that look like government mail. No federal agency sells long-term health insurance, nor does Medicare.

Your agent may be able to print out a proposed plan for you. My agent did this for me. The printout gave me a quick overview of the policy: yearly cost, daily maximum benefit, lifetime maximum benefit, and the benefit increase option.

I did not buy the insurance because it didn't mesh with our existing policies. Some health insurance plans allow for limited long-term care. Store all of the insurance paper—every scrap of paper and envelope—in a safe place. Tell family members where the papers are so they can find them in an emergency.

Working After Retirement

Many people want to work after they retire. Associated Press writer Alice Ann Love writes about work in her article, "Boomers Plan to Work in Retirement." Her article is based on a study conducted by the American Association of Retired Persons (AARP). A poll was taken at AARP's 40th anniversary convention in Minneapolis.

The telephone survey of 2001 Americans born between 1946 and 1964 showed that a third of these people want to work after they retire. Five percent said they plan to try an entirely new career. A surprising 17 percent of the survey respondents said they want to start their own businesses. "More than three-quarters admit to being more self-indulgent and needing more money to live comfortably than their parents," writes Love.

My husband and I are grappling with the work issue right now. We enjoy our jobs and, despite some health setbacks, want to work as long as possible. Lately, we have spent a lot of time discussing trade-offs, such as full-time and part-time work. Our retirement planning started with the basics:

- What state do we want to live in?
- What town do we want to live in?
- What kind of house do we want?
- What improvements will it need?
- What are our monthly expenses?
- Can we live happily on less?

Many of our friends are grappling with similar issues.

Sadly, age discrimination continues to be an issue in this country. National legislation has not eliminated the issue and older workers are still being forced out of their jobs.

Age Discrimination

Sara Czaja takes on age discrimination in her study, "Employment Opportunities for Older Adults: Engineering Design and Research Issues." American workers are supposed to be protected under the Age Discrimination Employment Act passed in 1967. The legislation may work in theory but not in practice. "Older workers are discriminated against in many ways; for example, they experience negative biases in performance ratings and are bypassed for promotion and retraining opportunities," writes Czaja.

Age discrimination is often subtle and that's why it is hard to prove. You may be excluded from planning meetings, for example. Being patronized, or in some instances, mistreated, by younger workers may be the most hurtful of all.

I was the oldest worker in a business office. Unfamiliar with computers at the time, I was constantly "kidded" by younger workers. They dazzled me with jargon and complained about the amount of paper I used. My work performance didn't stop their "kidding."

The boss had just left on a business trip when two workers approached my desk. "Before Ed (not the boss's real name) left he talked with us," one said. "We are the project managers now." Needless to say, the announcement surprised me. "I don't know anything about this," I replied.

The women looked so guileless, and we were on a tight deadline, so I believed them. Besides, I had plenty of other work to do. "I'll give you my files," I said.

After the incident my job lost its luster. Normally cheerful and outgoing, I became quiet and sullen at work. Maybe my mind was trying to tell me something. It turns out Ed had not removed me from the project and the whole thing was a sham.

Later, Ed called me into his office to discuss the incident. He praised my work and said my maturity had improved office dynamics. Flattery was no consolation, in my mind, especially since the women were never reprimanded.

I have often wondered what they wanted. Power? Prestige? A middle-aged mom? Perhaps I was their shortcut: I had done the research and they would get the credit. As cloudy as their purpose was, the message came through loud and clear: It's OK to trick honest, hard-working older employees.

About 17,000 cases of age discrimination are reported to the Equal Employment Opportunity Commission (EEOC) each year, according to Lisa Berger, author of Feathering Your Nest: The Retirement Planner. A measly 200 cases or less are taken to court. However, the news isn't all gloom and doom.

Massachusetts lets plaintiffs seek jury trials and doubles or triples damages in age discrimination cases. "The best weapon against age discrimination, say organizations that are fighting it, is individual testing," writes Berger.

Still, the time comes when you walk out the door. Before you leave, be sure to take advantage of any outplacement services that are available. These services may include resume writing, interviewing techniques, and access to computer databases. You may be able to use other office equipment as well, such as photocopiers and fax machines.

Outplacement Services

Journalist Carol Smith writes about outplacement services in her *Seattle Post-Intelligence* article, "Swedish Helps Its Employees Advance Toward Dream Jobs." Smith says outplacement services for laid-off workers are not new. But Swedish Medical Center started a plan to help employees find new positions inside and outside the organization.

The Employee Advancement Center offers Internet services, one-to-one counseling, and interview training. Employees use the center to focus their goals and make career plans. Director Robert Hamilton is quoted as saying "even if the goals are taking them away … as long as they're working toward a goal, they'll be more satisfied and productive while they're here."

Employees were skeptical about the Employment Advancement Center at first. Now the concept is catching on and 20 to 25 employees a week are using the services to find new jobs. Some of the jobs have been in-house. For example, a print shop employee moved up to the marketing department.

Other Seattle businesses are interested in the Employment Advancement Center model. One reason for their interest is the shortage of skilled labor. Older workers are filling the gap. As Carol Simpson reported on the *ABC Evening News,* "From service, to retail, to industry, older workers are in demand."

Demand for Older Workers

Melissa Levy describes the growing demand in her article, "Job Seniority." The unemployment rate in Minnesota was 3.2 percent when this book was written, and seems to be going lower. State businesses that want to expand "must turn to a group of workers they might not ordinarily court—older people."

Seniors are working for a variety of reasons, according to Levy:

- Boredom (no rocking on the front porch for these folks)
- Need (supplementing pensions and Social Security checks)
- Social stimulation (seniors like the day-to-day challenges of being on the job)
- Mental stimulation (older workers may have a variety of jobs with the same employer)
- Career change

"Some hope to embark on a second career without the corporate stress," explains Levy.

Walmart stores in Minnesota have made it a point to hire older workers. More than 10 percent of the Walmart employees in Minnesota, 9,151 of them to date, are over age 55. Levy notes that older people enjoy working in groups and trying jobs they haven't tried before.

By the year 2025 Minnesota's aging population is expected to increase 20 percent. Cynthia Cook saw the trend and started Retirement Enterprises in Bloomington, Minnesota, an employment service for older workers. Other agencies are focusing on older workers as well.

Finding Work

Finding a job in your later years can be a job itself. Word of mouth works best in my area. Call local employment agencies and ask if they have job listings for older workers. Check public bulletin boards for listings, too. Also contact:

- Your state senior career office, if one exists
- American Association of Retired Persons (AARP)
- National Council on Aging
- U.S. Department of Labor, Older Work Program

You will find the addresses for these organizations in the appendix.

As they near retirement many older workers think of becoming consultants. Think again. Lisa Berger, author of *Feathering Your Nest: The Retirement Planner,* says we should approach consulting work cautiously. It is one thing to call yourself a consultant, quite another thing to be one. "You'll need to market your services to local companies, a task that's no less daunting and demanding than job hunting," she writes.

If you can't find a job, you may want to move to another community. Adult children and grandchildren may factor into your decision. My husband and I have moved so many times we are moving experts. We're also tired of it. That's why we have decided to stay in the same house and adapt it to our needs.

Time to Move?

Is it time for you to move? Merril Silverstein, of the University of Southern California's Andrus Gerontology Center, studied moving patterns in the aging. His study, "Stability and Change in Temporal Distance Between the Elderly and Their Children," builds on data from a previous longitudinal study.

Silverstein says three events influence an older person's decision to move. The first move is due to retirement, maybe warmer weather, and an easier lifestyle.

The second move is due to the onset of physical and mental disabilities. The third move is usually to an institution, "after severe disability has put prohibitive demands on informal caregivers."

Time and travel costs may prompt family members to move closer to their aging relatives. The vulnerable aging may move closer to their children for support. Moving is costly and there are many things to consider beforehand.

MOVING CONSIDERATIONS

Ken Stern, a Certified Financial Planner, details the considerations in his article, "Smart Moves." "Realize that the best way to stretch your money is to plan ahead," he writes. Some key points to consider:

- Your personal comfort if your spouse dies
- Things for you to do in the area
- Things for your children and grandchildren to do
- State and local taxes
- Which is better, renting or buying?

- Available health care
- Transportation (private and public)

Stern says you need to decide whether this will be your primary or secondary home. Is this a good place for another career? Are there educational opportunities for you? Retired military people may want to look for a home near a base to take advantage of service benefits.

We may also learn from others. When my mother moved away from Long Island she made one of the greatest mistakes of her life. She left behind everything she had ever known: a house she loved, her circle of friends, the community church, and familiar stores and landmarks. From that time on Mom was lost.

Many of our friends have moved to the Southwest and urge us to move there. We visited the area several times and decided it wasn't for us. The cost of living was much higher, for one thing. Because of skin problems I am not supposed to be out in the sun. And neither of us tolerates the heat very well.

I have heard that a warm climate helps arthritis patients. If I had arthritis and had to move to the Southwest, I would probably do it. However, it would require a lot of emotional effort.

Do your homework before the van pulls up to the door. Pick out some locations and write the Chamber of Commerce for information. Visit for a week or two. Your research could save you time, disappointment, and money.

Retirement Communities

Some people enjoy community living and you may be one of them. Retirement communities come in many shapes and sizes, including: private home, townhouse, apartment, and high-rise. Jo Horne, author of *Caregiving: Helping an Aging Loved One,* details the advantages of "a structured setting."

Horne thinks services are the main advantage of retirement communities. These services may include transportation, utilities, cleaning, laundry, meal preparation, and an activities program.

Social networks are another advantage. As Horne explains, "For those who have become increasingly depressed and reclusive while living alone, such settings can provide the added advantage of opportunities for creative expression and social contact."

Giving up your home is hard to do, but it may be necessary. Moving to a retirement community doesn't mean you give up all independence. You can use the services when you want to and go your own way when you don't. Several of my friends live in a high-rise community and say they like the security it provides.

Contact the American Association of Retirement Communities for more information. The address is 2020 Pennsylvania Avenue, Suite 902, Washington, DC 20006. Or call 800-517-3847. Moving into a retirement community is a major change in your life—proof that you are older.

Turning Points

Life is not always smooth sailing and we all have times when we must make crucial choices. Bettyclare Moffatt, author of *Soulwork: Clearing the Mind, Opening the Heart, Replenishing the Spirit,* calls these times "turning points." When we are in the midst of a turning point—or crisis—we may feel paralyzed.

No matter how hard we try, we can't seem to move forward. Fighting the turning points saps our energy. What can we do? Moffatt says we can decide to trust life and let it take care of itself. "This process is not a 'giving up,' it is a 'letting go,'" she writes.

After our daughter's car crash, while she hovered near death, I was emotionally crushed. We had just emerged from 10 years of crisis and the crash was the final blow. Life had knocked me down and I didn't think I would get up again. "It's too much!" I cried, tears streaming down my face. "It's too much!" I was a nervous wreck and didn't know what to do.

Usually I get up at 5:30 A.M., but I started getting up 5:00 to meditate. We lived in the country then and I heard the countryside awaken. Birds singing. Leaves rustling. Distant cars. Total silence.

Ever so slowly, the answers to my questions seeped into my consciousness. I still meditate early in the morning. Bettyclare Moffatt might say I have developed a "listening soul." She describes the meditation process.

1. Words may come to mind.

2. No words may come to mind.

3. We may have a rush of feelings—even cry.

4. Finally, we encounter deep silence.

"Beyond that place is everything," writes Moffatt. I found the deep silence she describes and within that silence made a discovery. After all these years I am not afraid to fail. Because I am not afraid of failure I find more joy in life.

Each turning point alters life in some way. Positive outcomes may come from tragedy, although you may not be able to see them until time has passed. What are the turning points in your life? List them on page xx in the appendix and look for positive outcomes.

Turning points are not on your map but, like summer road work, you will encounter them. And you know what? Age is on your side. The turning points in life keep you from becoming complacent. You may find new towns, new friends, and new ideas, and call these places home.

Smart Aging Tips

⌒

- Track your monthly and yearly savings.

- Find out more about the retirement processes and procedures.

- Take advantage of the training programs where you work.

- Be aware of Economic Outpatient Care (EOC) and the reasons for it.

- Make a financial plan.

- Look into starting a college fund.

- Make a legal plan.

- Research long-term care insurance.

- Keep a list of your retirement needs and revise it when necessary.

- Make a financial plan for retirement.

- Look into post-retirement employment.

- Fight age discrimination.

- Contact local, state, and national groups about job opportunities after retirement.

- Do your moving homework.

- Visit retirement communities.

- Look for positive outcomes in the turning points of life.

9

Coming to Terms with Life

Coming to terms with life is an ongoing process and we confront many issues along the way. For most of us life span is the crucial issue. Just because my mother lived to the admirable age of 93 doesn't mean I will live that long.

Having a parent die forces us to deal with our own mortality. After both parents are gone the pattern of life becomes crystal clear: We are born, we live, and we die. Now we are next in line. "How long will I live?" we ask ourselves.

I don't know the answer, but I know I want to spend more time with my husband, watch our grandchildren grow, and make the most of my remaining years. The life spans of older people differ greatly. Life span is determined by a variety of factors, such as socioeconomic status.

How Long Will I Live?

Eileen Crimmins, MD, and her colleagues discuss longevity in their study, "Differentials in Active Life Expectancy in the Older Population of the United States." According to the researchers, "Current evidence on mortality and disability differences by education suggests that active life expectancy varies by socioeconomic status in much the same way as mortality."

Lower socioeconomic status also increases our chances of disability. Age and sex differences play a part in determining our longevity. While the gap is narrowing between the sexes, women still live longer than men, a fact well known to insurance companies. The researchers say "males across all levels of disability are more likely to die than females."

When my mother moved into her retirement community women outnumbered men and the average age of the residents was 86. Average may not mean what you think. Once you have passed a critical age, what is critical to your health, the chances of longevity increase. It's a statistical thing.

An increasing number of people, both older and younger, are slowing down to prolong their lives and improve the quality of their lives. Slowing down is a philosophy that requires thought, planning, and follow-through. How do you go about it?

Slowing Down

Richard Carlson and Joseph Bailey tell you how in their book, *Slowing Down to the Speed of Life*. They cite the reasons for slowing down. Obviously, slowing down reduces stress. Physical health also improves. Some other reasons for slowing down:

- Slowing down helps us to live in the present, or what some call "the moment"
- Slowing down heightens our awareness of life
- Slowing down gives us more peace of mind
- Slowing down helps us to be more creative and productive

We begin to slow down by becoming attuned to our feelings. As Carlson and Bailey write, "If you listen to these feelings and trust what they are trying to tell you, you will begin to experience the peace and joy of your mental health."

Smart Aging

Knowing our feelings and showing them are two different things. Showing your feelings in the workplace may be considered a sign of weakness, especially in women. Some people still think men are pragmatic and women are emotional. Managers want us to get our work done efficiently, with as little fuss as possible, and no "warm fuzzies," please.

Here is where the authors' concept of working smarter, not harder, comes into play. "Working smart implies listening, reflecting, and then acting rather than reacting out of habit," they explain. Fortunately, these attributes come with aging.

Last, Carlson and Bailey think we need to learn to empty our minds. They believe the mind needs sleep like the body needs sleep; "It needs to be empty, not in active use."

Emptying my mind is hard for me because I am a creative person and my mind goes in many directions at once. However, with lots of practice, I learned how to do it. I visualize a blank television screen. When a picture comes on the screen I blank it out. If I have trouble blanking it out I "color" the screen gray. This technique helps me to get back to sleep in the middle of the night.

Reading is another way I empty my mind. I divide my reading into "light" and "heavy." For some reason, and I don't know why, light reading clears my mind of junk.

Cookbooks fall into the light reading category and I read them the way some people read novels.

Working with my hands also helps to empty my mind. My father's bureau has been in the garage for months, covered with a sheet, waiting to be refinished. Soon I will tackle the job and, as I sand the wood, will think of him. Dad liked to refinish furniture, too; he varnished his boyhood desk and gave it to me.

You probably have other ways to empty your mind. Certainly, a rested mind is better at problem-solving. But some aging people are trying to solve their problems with risky behavior. In fact, risky behavior has become a worrisome national trend.

Risky Behavior

Journalist Monika Guttman examines the trend in her article, "The New Science of Risky Behavior." The article includes a chart of risky behavior:

- Poor diet
- Obesity
- Lack of regular dental care
- No leisure time/exercise
- Stress
- No sun protection
- Not wearing a seatbelt
- Smoking
- Alcohol abuse
- Sleep deprivation

People who engage in risky behavior have similar reasons for it; "magical thinking" is one of them. Their so-called reasoning: *It won't hurt me.* The reason is childlike in its simplicity and does not take logic, facts, or experience into account.

Genetics is also a reason for risky behavior. Often a form of denial, this reason gives the person tacit permission to continue with risky behavior. The risky behavior may escalate.

Need is another reason: one more cigarette, one more drink, one more gambling trip. Unfortunately, need may grow into bona fide addiction. Once addicted, it is hard to turn life around again.

Boredom, especially boredom after retirement, is yet another reason. I don't understand this reason because the world is filled with things to do. Nobody should be bored in this day and age.

Timing is the last reason. The people who cite this reason believe their lives are so busy they don't have time to change their behavior. "I'll get to it," they say. Many don't get to it, and risky behavior eventually puts their lives at risk.

Guttman explains, "This year, unhealthy behavior will account for 1 million deaths—nearly half of the total US deaths." The National Institutes of Health is so concerned about risky behavior it has joined forces with the American Heart Association to study the problem. Thirteen million dollars have been allocated for research.

Alcohol Abuse

A common theory says aging people drink because of stress.

Two researchers, J. W. Welte, PhD, and Amy Mirand, PhD, look at the theory in their study, "Drinking, Problem Drinking and Life Stressors in the Elderly General Population." They conducted a phone survey in Erie County, New York, and interviewed 2,325 people 60 years or older to see if stress influences late-onset drinking. The researchers defined a late-onset heavy drinker as someone who started drinking heavily after age 60, but not before that. Stress did not seem to play a part in late-onset heavy drinking. But the researchers discovered that chronic stress (as opposed to acute stress), is related to excess consumption.

Although excess consumption and heavy drinking are not defined, I can see a difference between the two. Heavy drinking tends to be ongoing behavior, whereas excess consumption is often sporadic—a New Year's party, for example. However, chronic stress can lead to heavy drinking and addiction.

If two people have consumed the same amount of alcohol, the researchers say, the person with the most chronic stress has the most dependence on alcohol and the most consequences. Why? "Chronic stress works to increase problems and symptoms, independently of the effect of alcohol consumption," according to the researchers.

Drug Abuse

Around middle-age we start to add up our life scores. How many successes? How many failures? How many almosts? Coming to terms with life is painful and some people abuse drugs to dull their pain. An article by Natalie Hopkinson, "Drug Use by Elderly an 'Epidemic,'" reports 17 percent of adults over age 60 are abusing drugs.

The numbers seem to be going up. Hopkinson says aging people may turn to drugs and alcohol after a significant life change, such as the death of a spouse. Caregivers may assume that confused patients are suffering from dementia, when the real problem is drug abuse.

Many baby boomers used recreational drugs. Experts think drug abuse in the aging will get even worse as the baby boomers age. Drugs and alcohol can be a deadly combination.

According to an Associated Press article, "Painkiller Overdose Can Damage Liver," acetaminophen can cause liver damage in alcoholics. When acetaminophen drugs, such as Tylenol and Excedrin, are combined with alcohol they are more toxic. Aging people may take drugs to promote sleep, and overdose accidentally. The symptoms of overdose are sweating, convulsions, yellow eyes, yellow skin, and diarrhea.

What can be done about drug and alcohol abuse? One solution is to limit intake. Doctors can screen their patients for abuse. Health care providers can educate people on the dangers of drugs and alcohol. Treatment is another option.

Brigid Schulte writes about the "Elderly Reclaiming Life After Alcoholism" in her Knight-Ridder Newspapers article. Nearly a fourth of all hospitalized people over the age of

60 are diagnosed with alcoholism, she reports. "Researchers estimate only 10 percent of those with alcohol problems make it through a [treatment] center's front door."

For more information on the treatment of alcohol and drug abuse call:

- National Council on Alcoholism and Drug Dependence, 800-622-2255

- National Drug and Alcohol Abuse and Treatment Referral Line, 800-662-4357

- Alcohol Treatment Referral Hotline, 800-ALCOHOL

- Hazelden Foundation, 800-1-DO-CARE (also treats gambling addiction)

- National Clearinghouse for Alcohol and Drug Information, 800-729-6686

As more states turn to gambling to make up for their financial shortfalls, more people are becoming addicted to gambling. News programs update viewers regularly on lottery jackpots. Some think these news spots are ads for gambling and foster a "get rich quick" mentality.

Addictive Gambling

Gambling became enough of a problem that the State Medical Society of Wisconsin published a series of articles about it in its journal. Jennifer Fessler wrote about aging people in her article, "Gambling Away the Golden Years."

Although there is meager research on gambling in the aging, Fessler says the anecdotal evidence is mounting, and older people "can be found in casinos all over the country at all hours of the day and night." The Wisconsin Addictions Board considers the state's elderly as the fastest growing population of addictive gamblers.

Often research statistics come from Gamblers Anonymous. But transportation problems and evening meetings keep many older people from attending the meetings, and they may not be represented in the statistics. Fessler says aging people gamble for a number of reasons.

Loneliness is one reason. The idea of flying to Las Vegas for a gambling weekend sounds exciting to a lonely person. The inactivity of retirement may lead to low self-esteem and gambling may be a way of dealing with this.

Some older people (and my mother was one of them) try to "earn" money by gambling. Mom had squandered my father's insurance money, about $200,000, and been defrauded of an additional $50,000. Her solution was to play the lottery. Needless to say, my mother never won anything, and losing money on the lottery made her more depressed.

"Depression, anxiety, marital and relationship troubles, and chemical dependency make some [aging people] more prone to becoming gambling addicts," writes Fessler.

Doctors may not pick up on gambling problems because it's unethical to ask a patient about finances. Addictive gamblers, like other addicts, are good at cover-ups. Experts are urging doctors to be aware of the symptoms of addiction: exhaustion, stress, depression, short attention span, sleep problems, weight loss, and isolation.

If a relative is abusing gambling, drugs, or alcohol, you might want to join Al Anon. The number should be in the business section of your phone book. Identify the risky behaviors in your life and avoid these detours, because they take you nowhere.

What Can't Be Changed?

In order to come to terms with life we must admit some things can't be changed. Maya Angelou writes about life's obstacles in her book, *Wouldn't Take Nothing for My Journey Now.* She quotes her grandmother, who said, "If you can't change it, change the way you think about it."

I had to change the way I thought about road development. The road that leads to our house divides city and county land. A plan to widen the road had been on the city books for a long time. We didn't pay much attention to the plan until the bulldozers came. Road construction took two years and the traffic patterns changed daily. We literally drove in circles. Usually a prompt person, I became a late person. When the road finally opened I breathed a sigh of relief.

My relief was short-lived. Work started on a new house next door and within weeks the vertical timbers were up, the house was enclosed, and windows were installed. Our view, a pioneer farm, weathered hills, and a winding country road, totally disappeared. Oh, there is a patch of sky in one corner of our window, and tree branches in the other, but the view is gone. "This has wounded my soul," I told my husband.

To make matters worse, the construction work frightened the wildlife away. We used to see as many as 16 deer grazing in the meadow below us. A large woodchuck lived behind the house. Bunnies snuggled in our woodpile for the winter. And hummingbirds buzzed by the deck. No more.

After some brainstorming sessions we decided to add more landscaping to our side yard. To do this, we had to remove a tree that was about to fall over. This made the rear corner of our property look better. The shadow of the new house provided us with more shade on the deck.

Instead of focusing on the negatives, I started focusing on the positives of the situation. The additional trees and shrubs give us something to enjoy as the seasons change. Other new homes on the cul de sac shield us from the highway. What things in your life can't be changed? Impossible as it sounds, you may be able to change your thinking about them.

What Can Be Changed?

Maya Angelou says she is finally comfortable inside her skin. I know what she means. Aging helps us to become comfortable with ourselves and to live well. She thinks the art of living well can be developed. You need:

- A love of life
- Ability to find pleasure in small things
- Realize that "the world owes you nothing"
- Accept gifts as gifts

"Living life as art requires a readiness to forgive," she writes in *Wouldn't Take Nothing for My Journey Now*. The opposites of forgiveness—grudges and scheming and aggression—are harmful to us. Our lives will be richer if we can forgive others.

Our lives will also be richer if we can cut out some of the stressors, or what I call hassle factors. Hassles are like bees; a few may sting you or you may be attacked by a swarm. The pace of modern life is a hassle in itself.

Hassle Factors

I don't know about the hassles in your life, but I can make some educated guesses. Here are some tips for eliminating hassles from your life.

CUT THE NOISE. Turn off the television, the radio, the CD player, and the beeper, and let quiet reign. You may be surprised at the thoughts you discover. In the quiet you may rediscover yourself.

PLAN THINKING TIMES. Every day should contain some thinking time. Your time may be early in the morning, like mine, or later on. Five minutes of reflection can get you through the day.

GET AWAY. You don't have to take an expensive vacation to get away. Take Friday or Monday off and have a mini vacation. If you can take a longer vacation, so much the better.

SAY NO. People try to get us to do things by playing on our sympathy and vanity. Don't fall for these tactics. Say no. The world will not come to an end because you have given a negative reply.

DO HOLIDAY SHOPPING YEAR-ROUND. The holidays have turned into a crowded marketing event. That's why I shop year-round. This spreads out the cost and I get in on summer sales and special mark-downs.

FIND HELP. The proverb, "Many hands make light work" is true. Divide tasks among family members or hire help, if necessary. My husband and I can't mow the lawn any more so we have a college student do it for us.

You will find other ways to cut the hassles from your life. An increasing number of Americans are joining the simplicity movement. Journalist Tom McNichol says the movement began in the 19th century with Henry Thoreau.

Simplify, Simplify, Simplify!

McNichol details the simple life in his article, "The Simplicity Movement: Living on Less and Liking It." Many Americans want to avoid "affluenza," he says, and are taking steps to do just that.

Before you simplify your life you must evaluate your finances. Would you share a home with another family to lower expenses? Could you take the bus to work? Will your children be financially secure?

In the last few years I have made a conscious effort to simplify my life. Yesterday I volunteered with many community groups. Today I volunteer with a few. At this stage of life I would rather do a few things well than many things poorly.

Clearing out stuff is another way to simplify life. Our rule: If we haven't used it in two years, we don't need it.

(The exception to the rule is our "historic" snow blower.) We give extra stuff to our children, the church rummage sale, and the Salvation Army.

We also believe in repairing items, such as our 20-year-old couch. The couch was the right scale for the family room, and since we liked the design, we had it recovered. Now the couch is as good as new and we have helped the environment.

Spirituality

An article in the *Mayo Clinic Women's HealthSource* says spirituality helps us to lead healthier lives. The Mayo Medical School, along with 30 other medical schools in the nation, offers courses in spirituality and healing. Some doctors are studying spirituality on their own.

The article says prayer, or meditation, "decreases muscle tension and lowers heart rate." A special insert describes intercessory prayers, a practice that is becoming more common in the medical community. To me, an ancient Sanskrit poem is like a prayer. It ends with the words, "Look to this day! For it is life." I say the words to myself in the morning. That I am alive is a miracle. Compared to the universe my life is a blip in time and I want to savor it.

I take care of my spiritual self. However, I don't think I have to go to church regularly to do this. Deep inside me there is a well of spirituality and I visit it often. Quiet, contemplative times help me to refill the well.

Family Stories

Long before electricity was invented families sat around and told stories. Columnist James Lileks writes about family stories in his article, "We Interrupt This Program for No Particular Reason." He tells about the death of his grandma-in-law, who died of "chronic mortality" at the age of 80.

Grandma gave all family members a sense of their Italian heritage. A fabulous cook and clothing store owner and manager, she took a gun along on buying trips. Although she didn't know how use it, Lileks exclaims, "Grandma packed a gat in the Big Apple!"

He thinks every family has stories to tell and says they are more interesting than slick magazine pieces. Because we are descended from second generation immigrants, my husband and I are both storytellers. This is not unusual. Immigrant families tell stories to retain a sense of family, to pass on skills, and to entertain each other.

My husband's family made their way from Illinois, up the Mississippi River, to Minnesota, where they became farmers. Every adult family member knows the story of the boy, Thomas Corrin Hodgson, and a relative who spent the winter in a 14- by 18-foot shanty. The pioneers lived on flour and water pancakes and fish from the river.

Eight months passed and the pioneers felt increasingly worse. They didn't know they had scurvy. An itinerant traveler, by his own account a doctor destroyed by drink, diagnosed their condition. He prescribed mustard plasters and fresh vegetables.

Later, Thomas Corrin Hodgson said the tramp doctor and his neighbors saved his life. I tell stories about my husband's family because my family history is murky, at best, and there are few records. The people who could fill in the gaps are all gone.

Storytelling is a way to preserve family history. It may also lead you to solutions. I used to tell stories about the communication problems I had with my mother. Friends gave me practical tips, I researched communication, and this led to a book.

Connect with Kids

Children are the balance wheel of life. My home town, Rochester, Minnesota, is home of the Mayo Clinic. One day, when I was feeling depressed, I went to the clinic and sat down in the pediatric waiting room. I watched children come and go.

A little girl had metal rods supporting her head. A little boy could barely walk. Dozens of children passed by and they were, for the most part, good-natured and cheerful. An hour later I was in tears. I decided to stop feeling sorry for myself and get going.

Children's laughter can also keep us going. My twin grandchildren didn't know I had a basement office until they were about four years old. "What's that?" they asked, pointing to the computer screen.

"That's my computer," I replied. "See the words on the screen? This is how I write books."

The twins burst out laughing. "Oh Grandma, you are so funny!" they exclaimed.

Connect with kids as you age. If there are no children in your extended family, go to places where you will see them: the park, the grocery store, and church. You could volunteer in a daycare or read to kids at the library.

Get the Deals

A friend and I were discussing the latest movies. "I'm not buying those discount tickets," she declared. "Those are for old folks." Well, I am not afraid to admit my age or to accept senior discounts.

One local department store gives seniors free coffee on Wednesdays and a 15 percent discount. Many restaurants have special menu items for seniors. Airline ticket books are another good deal. Avoiding the deals won't make us younger, so we might as well use them.

Senior Discounts

Age requirements may vary, but the deals are out there.

Joan Rattner Heilman tells about travel deals in her book *Unbelievably Good Deals and Great Adventures That You Absolutely Can't Get Unless You're Over 50*. She offers these travel tips:

- Check the fares before making travel plans
- Carry proof of age with you and ask for a discount
- Keep restrictions in mind (month, days, time, etc.)
- Compare senior discounts with other rates (there may be an airfare war)
- See if your discount applies to other family members

SeniorNet (low-cost computer training) is another good deal. Heilman describes SeniorNet as "a national nonprofit organization dedicated to building a community of computer-literate older adults." There are 115 learning centers nationwide and all are staffed by volunteers.

An individual membership in SeniorNet costs $35 the first year and $25 thereafter. Couples pay $40 the first year and $30 thereafter. To learn more about SeniorNet write 1 Kearny Street, San Francisco, CA 94108. You may also call 800-747-6848 or E-mail them at seniornet@aol.com.

Follow Your Dreams

Society has not been kind to the aging. But Matilda Riley, DSc, and John Riley, Jr., PhD, authors of "Age Integration and the Lives of Older People," think change is in the wind. Almost three decades have been added to the human life span and this is changing attitudes. The Rileys use statistics to support their theory.

More older people are enrolling in college courses. Roughly 1,000 colleges in this country have students over the age of 65. Work options for the aging have expanded. As they write, "Many people in their productive years will be productive assets, rather than burdens, on the economy."

Aging people have more potential now than at any time in history. I think aging is the process of becoming ourselves. It takes time to figure out who we are and what we do. Age gives us the ability—and opportunity—to follow our dreams.

Is there something you have wanted to do? There is no better time to turn your dreams into reality. My husband is a retired Air Force officer and his dream is to fly on a space available basis after he retires. I have two choices here: share the dream or stay home and worry.

I have decided to share his dream.

I have my own dreams as well. Art has always been a major part of my life and I plan to do more artistic things, such as take a computer graphics course. When we follow our dreams we are tapping our emotional intelligence.

Daniel Goleman, author of *Emotional Intelligence: Why It Can Matter More Than IQ,* thinks intelligence is multiple. "There is no magic number to the multiplicity of human talents." Aging may help you to discover your hidden talents.

An old adage says youth is wasted on the young. I don't want age to be wasted on the aging. All of us are living on borrowed time and we don't know how much is left in the account. So savor the gift of life. This life, this moment, will never come again.

This Life, This Moment

Only in middle-age did I understand the idea of living the moment. I learned that a moment can be the difference between death and life. A moment can be the difference between sorrow and joy. All it takes is a moment.

Biographer Richard Meryman includes a profound quote about the moment in his book, *Andrew Wyeth: A Secret Life.*

He describes the importance of the Olson family to the artist's work. The Olsons, sister and brother, were Wyeth's neighbors, and many of his paintings depict scenes in their home.

Christina Olson could not walk, and his painting of her crawling through the grass became an American image. Wyeth was impressed by her dignity. He observed Christina closely over the years, the shadow of her head, scooting a chair across the floor, filling the stove with wood. "There's a feeling that, yes, you're seeing something that is happening momentarily, but it's also a symbol of what always happened in Maine," he said. "The eternity of the moment."

Although we cannot predict life accurately, we can savor the eternity of the moment. Each human life is a journey, with a beginning, an ending—a cadence all its own. The journey takes us to charted and uncharted places. When it comes to life, we are all explorers.

Smart Aging Tips

- Accept your mortality and move on.
- Slow down to the real speed of your life.
- Find ways to work smarter, not harder.
- Learn how to empty your mind.
- Avoid risky behaviors: alcohol abuse, drug abuse, and addictive gambling.
- Try to accept the things that can't be changed.
- Change the things that can be changed.
- Cut out the hassles.
- Simplify your life.
- Stay in touch with your spirituality.
- Tell family stories.
- Connect with kids whenever possible.
- Get the deals.
- Follow your dreams.
- Savor the "eternity of the moment."

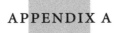

Tracking Your Turning Points

Review the turning points in your life, large and small, and write them here. List as many as possible.

_____

_____

_____

_____

_____

_____

_____

_____

_____

_____

_____

_____

_____

_____

_____

_____

_____

Look for the positive outcomes of your turning points. Write
the outcomes here.

_____

_____

_____

_____

_____

_____

_____

_____

_____

_____

_____

_____

_____

_____

_____

_____

_____

_____

_____

_____

_____

_____

_____

_____

_____

Helpful Associations and Agencies

Al-Anon Family Group Headquarters
1600 Corporate Landing Parkway
Virginia Beach, VA 23454
Phone: 757-563-1600
Fax: 757-563-1655

American Academy of Cosmetic Surgery
401 N. Michigan Avenue
Chicago, IL 60611-4212
Phone: 312-527-6713
Fax: 312-644-1815

American Academy of Dermatology
930 N. Meacham Road
Schaumburg, IL 60172-4965
Phone: 708-330-0230
Fax: 708-330-0050

American Aging Association
2129 Providence Avenue
Chester, PA 19013-5006
Phone: 610-874-7550
Fax: 610-876-7715

American Association of Retired Persons (AARP)
600 E Street NW
Washington, DC 20049
Phone: 800-4224-3410

American Association of Retirement Communities
2020 Pennsylvania Avenue, Suite 902
Washington, DC 20006
Phone: 800-517-3847

American Association of University Women (AAUW)
1111 16th Street NW
Washington, DC 20036-4873
Phone: 800-326-2289

American Dental Association
211 East Chicago Avenue
Chicago, IL 60611-2678
Phone: 800-621-8099

American Medical Association
515 North Lake Street
Chicago, IL 60610
Phone: 800-458-5736

American Savings Education Council
2121 K Street NW, Suite 600
Washington, DC 20037-1896
Internet: http://www.asec.org

American Society for Geriatric Dentistry
211 East Chicago Avenue, Suite 948
Chicago, IL 60611
Phone: 312-440-2661
Fax: 312-440-2824

Better Hearing Institute
Box 1840
Washington, DC 20013
Phone: 703-642-0580
Fax: 703-750-9302

Elderhostel Institute Network
75 Federal Street
Boston, MA 02112-1941
Phone: 617-426-7788

Environmental Alliance for Senior Involvement
8733 Old Dumfries Road
Catlett, VA 20119
Phone: 540-788-3274

Five Wishes Living Will
PO Box 11180
Tallahassee, FL 32302-3180
Phone: 850-681-2010
Fax: 850-681-2481
Internet: http://www.agingwithdignity.org

Food and Drug Administration (FDA)
5600 Fishers Lane, Parklawn Building
Rockville, MD 20857
Phone: 301-443-3170
800-332-4010

Habitat for Humanity International
1511 K Street NW, #605
Washington, DC 20005
Phone: 202-628-9171
Fax: 202-628-9169

Hazelden Foundation
15245 Pleasant Valley Road
PO Box 11
Center City, MN 55012-0011
Phone: 612-257-4010
Fax: 612-257-5101

Learn and Serve America (Corporation for National Service)
1201 New York Avenue NW
Washington, DC 20525
Phone: 800-942-2677
Fax: 202-565-2787

Library of Congress
10 1st Street SE
Washington, DC 20540
Phone: 202-707-5522 (General reference)
202-707-6400 (Recorded information)
Fax: 202-707-5844

Narcotic Educational Foundation of America
24509 Walnut Street, Suite 201
Santa Clarita, CA 91321-2846
Phone: 805-287-0198

National Alliance of Senior Citizens
1744 Riggs Place NW, 3rd floor
Washington, DC 20009-2508
Phone: 202-986-0117
Fax: 202-986-2974

National Association of Insurance Commissioners
120 W. 12th Street, Suite 1100
Kansas City, MO 64105-1925
Phone: 816-842-3600

National Council on Aging
409 3rd Street SW
Washington, DC 20024
Phone: 202-479-1200

National Institutes of Health
1 Center Drive, Building 1, #126
Bethesda, MD 20892-0148
Phone: 301-496-2433
Fax: 301-402-2700

National Park Service
Department of the Interior Building, Room 3104
Washington, DC 20013-7127
Phone: 202-208-4621

Points of Light Foundation
1737 H Street NW
Washington, DC 20006
Phone: 202-223-9186
Fax: 202-223-9256

Retired and Senior Volunteer Program (Foster Grandparent Program, Senior Companion Program)
1201 New York Avenue NW
Washington, DC 20525
Phone: 800-972-2677
Fax: 202-656-2789

SeniorNet
1 Kearny Street
San Francisco, CA 94108
Phone: 800-747-6848
E-mail: seniornet@aol.com

Service Corps of Retired Executives (SCORE)
409 3rd Street SW, 4th floor
Washington, DC 20024
Phone: 202-205-6762

US Department of Labor (Senior Community Service Employment Program)
200 Constitution Avenue, Room N-4641
Washington, DC 20210
Phone: 202-219-5904

Volunteers of America
3939 North Causeway Boulevard
Metairie, LA 70002
Phone: 504-834-5243

APPENDIX C

Bibliography

ABC Good Morning America, June 16, 1998, information on 98-year-old high school graduate Cyrena Wooster.

ABC World News Tonight, April 20, 1998, information on Viagra.

ABC World News Tonight, September 30, 1997, "About Men" series.

Alzheimer's Association. "Estrogen and Alzheimer's Disease," *Advances: Progress in Alzheimer Research and Care* (newsletter), summer 1998, p. 2.

Anderson, Kjeld V. and Bovim, Gunnar. "Impotence and Nerve Entrapment in Long Distance Amateur Cyclists," *Acta Neyrologica Scandinavica,* 1997, pp. 233–240.

Anderson, Mary, DDS. "Portrait of Aging Teeth," *Discover* (published by Health Partners, Minneapolis, MN), summer 1993, pp. 10–11.

Angelou, Maya. *Wouldn't Take Nothing for My Journey Now.* New York: Bantam Books, 1997, pp. 47, 54–55.

Associated Press. "Painkiller Overdose Can Damage Liver," *Rochester Post-Bulletin,* October 16, 1997, p. 6A.

Associated Press. "Seniors Seeking Friends and Fitness on a Roll With Skating," *Minneapolis Star Tribune,* September 28, 1997, p. B2.

Associated Press. "Standards on Labeling Foods as Organic Released Today," *Rochester Post-Bulletin,* December 15, 1997, p. 8A.

Bachmann, Gloria A., MD. "Influence of Menopause on Sexuality," *International Journal of Fertility and Menopausal Studies,* Supplement 1, 1995, pp. 16–22.

Barry, Henry C., MD., and Eathorne, Scott W., MD. "Exercise and Aging: Issues for the Practitioner," *Medical Clinics of North America,* March 1994, pp. 357–376.

Beacham, Bruce E., MD. "Common Dermatoses in the Elderly," *American Family Physician,* May 1, 1993, pp. 1445–1450.

Beers, Mark H., MD., and Urice, Stephen K., PHD, JD. *Aging in Good Health.* New York: Pocket Books, 1992, pp. 18–19.

Berger, Lisa. *Feathering Your Nest: The Retirement Planner.* New York: Workman Publishing, 1993, pp. 24–29, 416–421.

Berkey, Douglas B., DMD, MPH, MS. "Geriatric Dentistry at the Crossroads," *Journal of Dental Education,* December 1996, pp. 939–942.

Biehl, Bobb. *Mentoring: Confidence in Finding a Mentor and Becoming One.* Nashville: Broadman & Holman Publishers, 1996, pp. 11–14.

Birge, Stanley J., MD. "Is There a Role for Estrogen Replacement Therapy in the Prevention and Treatment of Dementia?" *Journal of the American Geriatrics Society,* July 1996, pp. 865–879.

Blumberg, Dr. Jeffrey B. "The Requirement for Vitamins in Aging and Age-Associated Degenerative Conditions," *Bibliotheca Nutritio et Dieta,* 1995, pp. 108–115.

Bonnet, Michael H., PHD, and Arand, Donna L. "We Are Chronically Sleep Deprived," *Sleep,* December 1995, pp. 908–911.

Bosse, Raymond, et al. "Change in Social Support After Retirement: Longitudinal Findings From the Normative Aging Study," *Journal of Gerontology,* July 1993, pp. 210–217.

Boston Globe. "We're Living Longer—And Better," article published in the *Rochester Post-Bulletin,* October 17, 1997, p. 2A.

Brody, Jane E. "Supplement Use is Unregulated Minefield," *New York Times* News Service article published in the *Minneapolis Star Tribune,* September 27, 1998, p. E5.

Brody, Jane E. "Study: Folate, B-6 May be Heart Healthy," *New York Times* News Service article published in the *Rochester Post-Bulletin,* February 4, 1998, p. 7A.

Brown, Jeff. "College-Age Kids, Retirement Budget," Knight Ridder Newspaper article published in the *Rochester Post-Bulletin,* July 11, 1998, pp. 1E.

Bruce, Martha Livingston, PHD, MPH, et al. "The Impact of Depressive Symptomatology on Physical Disability: MacArthur Studies of Successful Aging," *American Journal of Public Health,* November 1994, p. 1796–1799.

Buchowski, Maciej S., PhD, and Sun, Ming, PhD, "Nutrition Problems in Minority Elders: Current Problems and Future Directions," *Journal of Health Care for the Poor and Underserved,* August 1996, pp. 184–209.

Butler, Robert N., MD. "Living Longer, Contributing Longer," *Journal of the American Medical Association (JAMA),* October 22–29, 1997, pp. 1372–1373.

Carlson, Richard, PhD, *Don't Sweat the Small Stuff... And It's All Small Stuff.* New York: Hyperion, 1997, pp. 67–68, 141–142, 169–170.

Carlson, Richard, and Bailey, Joseph. *Slowing Down to the Speed of Life.* San Francisco: HarperSanFrancisco, 1997, pp. 4–5, 54–56, 69, 143, 157–158, 206.

Carman, Mary B., PhD, "The Psychology of Normal Aging," *The Psychiatric Clinics of North America,* March 1997, pp. 15–24.

Carnahan, Heather, et al. "The Influence of Summary Knowledge of Results and Aging on Motor Learning," *Research Quarterly for Exercise and Sport,* September 1996, pp. 280–287.

Casper, Regina C. "Nutrition and its Relationship to Aging," *Experimental Gerontology,* May-August 1995, pp. 299–314.

Chaplin, James P., PhD, *Dictionary of Psychology.* New York: Bantam Doubleday Dell Publishing Group, Inc., 1985, p. 416.

Chernoff, Ronni, PhD, RD. "Effects of Age on Nutrient Requirements," *Clinics in Geriatric Medicine,* November 1995, pp. 641–651.

Cole, Thomas R. and Winkler, Mary G., co-editors. *The Oxford Book of Aging.* New York: Oxford University Press, 1994, p. 323.

Coleman, Brenda. "Monitor Spots 'White-Coat Hypertension,'" Associated Press article published in the *Rochester Post-Bulletin,* November 10, 1997, p. 1D.

"Colon Cancer Screening," *Mayo Clinic Health Letter,* May 1992, pp. 1–4.

Crimmins, Eileen M., et al. "Differentials in Active Life Expectancy in the Older Population of the United States," *Journals of Gerontology,* May 1996, pp. S111-S120.

Czaja, Sara J. "Employment Opportunities for Older Adults: Engineering Design and Research Issues," *Experimental Aging Research,* October-December, 1994, pp. 265–273.

Dreyfuss, Ira. "Women Reduce Their Risk of Colon Cancer Through Exercise," Associated Press article published in the *Rochester Post-Bulletin,* July 28, 1997, p. 1D.

Ekstrom, Ireta, MEd. "Printed Materials for an Aging Population: Design Considerations," *Journal of Biocommunication,* Volume 20, Number 3, 1993, pp. 25–30.

Elder, Glen H. and Pavalko, Eliza K. "Work Careers in Men's Later Years: Transitions, Trajectories, and Historical Change," *Journal of Gerontology,* July 1993, pp. S180-S191.

Elderhostel United States Catalog, Fall 1998, p. 2.

Estrin, Robin. "'Grandfamilies House' Fills a Need," Associated Press article published in the *Rochester Post-Bulletin,* August 7, 1997, p. 4A.

"Exercise As You Age," *Medical Essay* (supplement to the *Mayo Clinic Health Letter*), February 1997, pp. 1–8.

"Exercise Equipment," *Mayo Clinic Health Letter,* September 1992, pp. 6–7.

Ezell, Hank. "Retirement Planning: Most of Us Way Behind," Cox News Service article in the *Rochester Post-Bulletin,* October 18, 1997, p. 1E.

Fessler, Jennifer L. "Gambling Away the Golden Years," *Wisconsin Medical Journal,* September 1996, pp. 618–619.

Foveaux, Jessie Lee Brown. *Any Given Day: A Memoir of Twentieth Century America.* New York: Warner Books, 1997, pp. 280.

Friedman, David, Dr., et al. "Implicit Retrieval Processes in Cued Recall: Implications for Aging Effects in Memory," *Journal of Clinical and Experimental Neuropsychology,* December 1994, pp. 921–938.

Galanis, Daniel J., et al. "Smoking History in Middle Age and Subsequent Cognitive Performance in Elderly Japanese-American Men," *American Journal of Epidemiology,* March 1997, pp. 507–515.

Galanos, Anthony N., MD, et al. "The Comprehensive Assessment of Community Dwelling Elderly: Why Functional Status Is Not Enough," *Aging,* October 1994, pp. 343–352.

Gale, Elaine. "The Dean of Writers," *Minneapolis Star Tribune,* July 20, 1997, pp. F1, F6.

Goldstein, Marion Zucker, MD, and Perkins, Cathy Ann, MD. "Mental Acuity and the Aging Woman," *Clinics in Geriatric Medicine,* February 1993, pp. 191–196.

Goleman, Daniel. *Emotional Intelligence: Why It Can Matter More Than IQ.* New York: Bantam Books, 1997, pp. 38–39, 90–91.

Goode, Stephen. "Sense and Sensibility," *Insight,* August 18, 1997, pp. 8–10.

Goodman, Ellen. "Meno—The Pause That Refreshes," syndicated article in the *Rochester Post-Bulletin,* October 7, 1997, p. 11A.

Gorbein, Martin J., MD. "When Your Older Patient Can't Sleep: How to Put Insomnia to Rest," *Geriatrics,* September 1995, pp. 65–73.

Gorman, Warren F., MD, and Campbell, Cris D., JD. "Mental Acuity of the Normal Elderly," *Journal of the Oklahoma State Medical Association,* March 1995, pp. 119–123.

Guttman, Monika. "The New Science of Risky Behavior," *USA Weekend,* March 6–8, 1998, pp. 4–5.

Haddy, Francis J., MD, PhD, et al. "Role of Dietary Salt in Hypertension," *Journal of the American College of Nutrition,* October 1995, pp. 428–438.

Hannien, Tuomo, MA, et al. "Subjective Memory Complaints and Personality Traits in Normal Elderly Subjects," *Journal of the American Geriatrics Society,* January 1994, pp. 1–4.

Heaney, Robert P., MD. "Age Considerations in Nutrient Needs for Bone Health: Older Adults," supplement to the *Journal of the American College of Nutrition,* December 1996, pp. 575–578.

Heilman, Joan Rattner. *Unbelievably Good Deals and Adventures That You Absolutely Can't Get Unless You're Over 50.* Chicago: Contemporary Books, 1998, pp. 7–8, 236.

Helfand, Arthur E., DPM. "Assessment of the Geriatric Patient," *Clinics in Podiatric Medicine and Surgery,* January 1993, p. 47–57.

Hellman, Esther A., MS, RN, and Stewart, Cynthia, PhD, RN. "Social Support and the Elderly Client," *Home Healthcare Nurse,* September-October 1994, pp. 51–60.

Hendren, John. " 'Wand' Waves the Pain Away from Dentists' Injections," *Rochester Post-Bulletin,* October 17, 1997, p. 2A.

Hillengass, Debbie, director of Distance Education, University of Minnesota, phone interview on June 29, 1998.

Holliman, Billie J., PharmD, and Chyka, Peter A., PharmD. "Problems of Assessment of Acute Melatonin Overdose," *Southern Medical Journal,* April 1997, pp. 451–453.

Holzapfel, Stephen, MD, CCFP. "Aging and Sexuality," *Canadian Family Physician,* April 1994, pp. 748–766.

Hopkinson, Natalie. "Drug Use by Elderly an 'Epidemic.'" Cox News Service article in the *Rochester Post-Bulletin,* May 8, 1998, p. 7A.

Horne, Jo. *Caregiving: Helping an Aging Loved One.* Glenview, Ill: Scott Foresman and Company, 1985, pp. 65–66.

Husted, Amanda. "Many Women Avoid Two Tests That Could Save Their Lives," Cox News Service article published in the *Rochester Post-Bulletin,* November 10, 1997, p. 1D.

Jacobs, Ruth Harriet, PhD, *Be an Outrageous Older Woman.* New York: Harper Collins, 1997, pp. 131–157.

Kaiser, Fran E., MD. "Sexuality in the Elderly," *Urologic Clinics of North America,* February 1996, pp. 99–109.

Keithley, Joyce K., DNSC, RN, FAAN. "Promoting Good Nutrition: Using the Food Guide Pyramid in Clinical Practice," *MEDSURG Nursing,* December 1996, pp. 397–403.

Kendler, Barry S., PhD, "Melatonin: Media Hype or Therapeutic Breakthrough?" *Nurse Practitioner,* February 1997, pp. 66–77.

Kendrick, Zebulon V., PhD, et al. "Metabolic and Nutritional Considerations for Exercising Older Adults," *Comprehensive Therapy,* 1994, pp. 558–568.

Kruger, Pamela. "Baby Boomers Find Themselves Unprepared for High Cost of College," *New York Times* News Service article in the *Minneapolis Star Tribune,* March 22, 1998, pp. D1-D4.

Lebowitz, Barry D., PhD, et al. "Diagnosis and Treatment of Depression in Late Life," *Journal of the American Medical Association (JAMA),* October 8, 1997, pp. 1186–1190.

Levine, Bettijane. "They've Got That Old Feeling: The Giddy Thrill of New Love," *Los Angeles Times* article published in the *Minneapolis Star Tribune,* August 24, 1997, p. E4.

Levy, Melissa. "Job Seniority," *Minneapolis Star Tribune,* October 5, 1997, pp. D1, D4.

Lileks, James. "We Interrupt This Program for No Particular Reason," *Minneapolis Star Tribune,* September 7, 1997, p. B3.

Lindoo, Susan, program director, Compleat & Practical Scholar program, University of Minnesota, phone interview on June 30, 1998.

Love, Alice Ann. "Boomers Plan to Work in Retirement," Associated Press article in the *Rochester Post-Bulletin,* June 2, 1998, p. 1.

Lyon, Jeff. "Amazing Medical Breakthroughs," *Family Circle,* October 7, 1997, pp. 83–84, 90, 92, 96, 98–99.

Maxson, Pamela, et al. "Multidimensional Patterns of Aging: A Cluster-Analytic Approach," *Experimental Aging Research,* January–March 1997, pp. 13–31.

Mayo Clinic. "Checkups: A Time for Action," *Mayo Clinic Women's HealthSource,* August 1997, p. 6

Mayo Foundation for Medical Education and Research. "Calcium," *Mayo Clinic Health Letter,* May 1995, pp. 4–5.

Mayo Foundation for Medical Education and Research. "Colon Cancer Screening," *Mayo Clinic Health Letter,* May 1992, pp. 1–4.

Mayo Foundation for Medical Education and Research. "Diagnostic Ultrasound," *Mayo Clinic Health Letter,* April 1992, pp. 4–5.

Mayo Foundation for Medical Education and Research. "Exercise Equipment," *Mayo Clinic Health Letter,* September 1992, pp. 6–7.

Mayo Foundation for Medical Education and Research. "Incontinence: Ways to Help You Stay Dry," *Mayo Clinic Health Letter,* January 1998, pp. 1–3.

Mayo Foundation for Medical Education and Research. "Mammograms: When to Start Screening," *Mayo Clinic Women's HealthSource,* February 1997, p. 6.

Mayo Foundation for Medical Education and Research. "Prostate Gland Enlargement," *Mayo Clinic Health Letter,* July 1992, pp. 4–5.

Mayo Foundation for Medical Education and Research. "Prostate Gland Enlargement: Treatment Options Grow," *Mayo Clinic Health Letter,* May 1996, pp. 1–3.

Mayo Foundation for Medical Education and Research. "Spirituality and Healing: Your Faith is Working in Your Favor," *Mayo Clinic Women's HealthSource,* July 1998, p. 7.

Mayo Foundation for Medical Education and Research. "The Vitamin Controversy," *Mayo Clinic Women's Health Source,* September 1998, pp. 1–2.

McNichol, Tom. "The Simplicity Movement: Living on Less and Liking It," *USA Weekend,* July 19–21, pp. 4–5.

Merrill, Ann. "Bridging the Generations," *Minneapolis Star Tribune,* September 21, 1997, pp. 1D, 4D.

Meryman, Richard. *Andrew Wyeth: A Secret Life.* New York: Harper Collins, 1996, pp. 12–13.

Mickley, Jacqueline Ruth, PhD, RN, et al. "Religion and Adult Mental Health: State of the Science in Nursing," *Issues in Mental Health Nursing*, July-August 1995, pp. 345–360.

Moffatt, Bettyclare. *Soulwork: Clearing the Mind, Opening the Heart, Replenishing the Spirit.* Berkeley: Wildcat Canyon Press, 1994, pp. 13–14, 26–27, 60, 152.

Murphy, Dr. Claire. "Nutrition and Chemosensory Perception in the Elderly," *Critical Reviews in Food Science and Nutrition,* January 1993, pp. 3–15.

National Association of Insurance Companies. *A Shopper's Guide to Long-Term Care Insurance* (booklet). Kansas City: National Association of Insurance Commissioners, 1986, pp. 4–6, 11, 15–17.

Neergaard, Lauran. "FDA Panel Recommends Osteoporosis Drug," Associated Press article in the *Rochester Post-Bulletin,* November 21, 1997, p. 1.

Neergaard, Lauran. "Impotence Pill Gains Approval," Associated Press article in the *Rochester Post-Bulletin,* March 28, 1998, p. 5A.

Neergaard, Lauran. "Test Helps Diagnose Thin Bones," Associated Press article in the *Rochester Post-Bulletin,* March 14, 1998, p. 8A.

Neporent, Liz. "Living-Room Leg Lifts: A Guide to TV Exercise Shows," *Good Housekeeping,* April 1998, pp. 59–60.

Nestle, Marion. "Food Lobbies, the Food Pyramid, and US Nutrition Policy," *International Journal of Health Services,* 1993, pp. 483–496.

New York Times News Service. "Patients Over 60 Are Cautioned on Painkillers," *Rochester Post-Bulletin,* July 28, 1997, p. 3D.

NIH Consensus Development Panel on Impotence. "Impotence," *Journal of the American Medical Association,* July 1993, pp. 83–90.

O'Hara, Delia. "Osteoporosis," *American Medical News,* October 6, 1997, pp. 12–15, 18.

Ott, A., PhD, et al. "Smoking and Risk of Dementia and Alzheimer's Disease in a Population-Based Cohort Study: The Rotterdam Study," *The Lancet,* June 20, 1998, pp. 1840–1843.

Paganini-Hill, Annlia. "Estrogen Replacement Therapy in the Elderly," *Zentralblatt für Gynakologie,* May 1996, pp. 255–261.

Painter, Kim. "New Calcium Advice: Eat More," *USA Today,* August 14, 1997, pp. 1, 8D.

Palmer, Mary E., MD. "Dietary Supplements: 'Natural' is not Always Safe," *Emergency Medicine,* September 1998, pp. 52–74.

Pearson, Jay D., et al. "Gender Differences in a Longitudinal Study of Age-Associated Hearing Loss," *Journal of the Acoustical Society of America,* February 1995, pp. 1196–1205.

Pickering, Thomas G., MD, DPhil. "A New Role for Ambulatory Blood Pressure Monitoring?" *Journal of the American Medical Association (JAMA),* October 1, 1997, p. 1110.

Prinz, Dr. Patricia N. "Sleep and Sleep Disorders in Older Adults," *Journal of Clinical Neurophysiology,* March 1995, pp. 139–146.

Reinhart, Theodora J., technical chairman. *ASM International Manual* 1993, p. 18.

Riley, Matilda White, DSc, and Riley, John W., Jr., PhD, "Age Integration and the Lives of Older People," *The Gerontologist,* February 1994, pp. 110–115.

Rimm, Eric B., ScD, et al. "Folate and Vitamin B6 from Diet and Supplements in Relation to Risk of Coronary Heart Disease Among Women," *Journal of the American Medical Association (JAMA),* February 4, 1998, pp. 359–364.

Ritter, Malcom. "Fix Your Face: More and More Men Removing Bags, Sags," Associated Press article in the *Rochester Post-Bulletin,* December 15, 1997, p. 2C.

Roenigk, Henry H., Jr., MD. "The Place of Laser Resurfacing Within the Range of Medical and Surgical Skin Resurfacing Techniques," *Seminars in Cutaneous Medicine and Surgery,* September 1996, pp. 208–213.

Russell, Robert M. and Suter, Paolo M. "Vitamin Requirements of Elderly People: An Update," *American Journal of Clinical Nutrition,* July 1993, pp. 4–14.

Schiavi, Raul C., MD, and Rehman, Jamil, MD. "Sexuality and Aging," *Urologic Clinics of North America,* November 1995, pp. 711–726.

Schiffman, Susan S., PhD. "Taste and Smell Losses in Normal Aging and Disease," *Journal of the American Medical Association (JAMA),* October 22, 1997, pp. 1357–1362.

Schow, Douglas A., MD, et al. "Male Menopause: How to Define It, How to Treat It," *Postgraduate Medicine,* March 1997, pp. 62–79.

Schuett, Dawn. "Courting the 'Golden Years,'" *Rochester Post-Bulletin,* March 21, 1998, p. 1B.

Schuett, Dawn. "Seniors Put a New Spin on Dating," *Rochester Post-Bulletin,* March 21, 1998, p. 6B.

Schulte, Brigid. "Elderly Reclaiming Life After Alcoholism," Knight-Ridder Newspapers article in the *Rochester Post-Bulletin,* January 12, 1998, p. 1C.

Sexton, Connie Cone. "60 and Still Going," *Arizona Republic,* October 14, 1997, pp. C1-C2.

Shay, Kenneth, DDS, MS, and Ship, Jonathan A., DMD. "The Importance of Oral Health in the Older Patient," *Journal of the American Geriatrics Society,* September 1996, pp. 1414–1422.

Shockman, Luke. "Ulcers an Easy Target," *Rochester Post-Bulletin,* August 21, 1997, p. 3A.

Silverstein, Merril. "Stability and Change in Temporal Distance Between the Elderly and Their Children," *Demography,* February 1995, pp. 29–45.

Simpson, Carol. ABC Evening News, February 10, 1998.

Skoe, Eva E., et al. "The Ethic of Care: Stability Over Time, Gender Differences, and Correlates in Mid-to-Late Adulthood," *Psychology and Aging,* June 1996, pp. 280–292.

Sloane, Philip D., MD, MPH. "Evaluation and Management of Dizziness in the Older Patient," *Clinics in Geriatric Medicine,* November 1996, pp. 785–801.

Smith, Carol. "Swedish Helps Its Employees Advance Toward Dream Jobs," *Seattle Post-Intelligence,* May 15, 1998, p. B1.

Smith, Lynn. "To Grandmother's House They Go," *Good Housekeeping,* February 1998, pp. 92–95.

Smoking Cessation Clinical Practice Guideline Panel and Staff. "The Agency for Health Care Policy and Research Smoking Cessation Clinical Practice Guideline," *Journal of the American Medical Association (JAMA),* April 24, 1996, pp. 1278–1279.

Snyderman, Nancy, MD. "Colon Cancer: Stopping a Killer in Our Midst," *Good Housekeeping,* September 1997, p. 58.

Solomon, Renee, DSW, and Peterson, Monte, MD. "Successful Aging: How to Help Your Patients Cope With Change," *Geriatrics,* April 1994, pp. 41–47.

"Spells," *Mayo Clinic Health Letter,* August 1997, pp. 1–3.

Springer, Ilene. "Health Alert! Drugs That Don't Mix," special insert, *Family Circle,* September 16, 1997, no page numbers.

Staff writer. "Herbal Roulette," *Consumer Reports,* November 1995, pp. 698–705.

Staff writer, "Myths About Mental Illness," *Menninger Perspective*, Number 2, 1997, pp. 25–29.

Stamatiadis, Nikiforos and Deacon, John A. "Trends in Highway Safety: Effects of an Aging Population on Accident Propensity," *Accident Analysis and Prevention*, August 1995, pp. 443–459.

Stanley, Thomas J., PhD, and Danko, William D., PhD, *The Millionaire Next Door*, Atlanta: Longstreet Press, 1996, pp. 142–143, 148.

Stern, Ken, Certified Financial Planner. "Smart Moves," *The Retired Officer*, September 1997, pp. 39–46.

Stevens, Joseph C. and Cain, William S. "Changes in Taste and Flavor in Aging," *Critical Reviews in Food Science and Nutrition*, January 1993, pp. 27–37.

Swift, Cameron G. and Shapiro, Colin M. "ABC of Sleep Disorders: Sleep and Sleep Problems in Elderly People," *British Medical Journal*, May 29, 1993, pp. 1468–1471.

Taylor, Allen et al. "Relations Among Aging, Antioxidant Status, and Cataract," *American Journal of Clinical Nutrition*, December 1995, pp. 1439S-1447S.

Taylor, Mary Anne and Shore, Lynn McFarlane. "Predictors of Planned Retirement Age: An Application of Beehr's Model," *Psychology and Aging*, March 1995, pp. 76–83.

Thiboutot, Diane M., MD. "Acne Rosacea," *American Family Physician*, December 1994, pp. 1691–1697.

"3M Employees Gather to Celebrate Dental Products' Achievement," *3M Stemwinder*, December 24, 1997, pp. 1, 15.

Tillotson, Kristin. "When We Appraise our Assets, Gray Matters," *Minneapolis Star-Tribune*, July 13, 1997, pp. F1, F10.

Tower, Kristine D. "Consumer-Centered Social Work Practice: Restoring Client Self-Determination," *Social Work*, March 1994, pp. 194–195.

Towey, James H., President, Commission on Aging With Dignity. Letter dated September 1997.

Towey, James H., President, Commission on Aging With Dignity, Today Show, NBC Television, August 14, 1997.

Turney, Lawrence M., Junior, MD. McPhee, Stephen J., MD. Papadakis, Maxine, AMD, editors. 1998 *Current Medical Diagnosis & Treatment.* Stamford: Appleton & Lange, 1998, pp. 339, 905.

University of Minnesota. *The Compleat & Practical Scholar* (newspaper). Minneapolis: University College, University of Minnesota, Spring 1998, p. 2.

University of Minnesota. *The Master of Liberal Studies* (brochure). Minneapolis: University College, University of Minnesota, no date.

Vowels, Darlene (American Association of University Women speaker) October 2, 1997.

Vuori, Ilkka. "Exercise and Physical Health: Musculoskeletal Health and Functional Capabilities," *Research Quarterly for Exercise and Sport,* December 1995, pp. 276–285.

Wellman, Nancy S., PhD, RD. "Dietary Guidance and Nutrient Requirements of the Elderly," *Primary Care: Clinics in Office Practice,* March 1994, pp. 1–18.

 Welte, J.W., PhD, and Mirand, Amy L., PhD, "Drinking, Problem Drinking and Life Stressors in the Elderly General Population," *Journal of Studies on Alcohol,* January 1995, pp. 67–73.

West, Maureen. "Lifetime of Habits Determines Differences in the Aging Process," *New York Times* News Service article printed in the *Rochester Post-Bulletin,* November 17, 1997, p. 1C.

Whelton, Paul K., MD, MSC, et al. "Sodium Reduction and Weight Loss in the Treatment of Hypertension in Older Persons," *Journal of the American Medical Association (JAMA),* March 18, 1998, pp. 839–846.

Wickre, Earlene, Coordinator of Business Services, Rochester, Minnesota Public Schools, phone interview on October 13, 1997.

Wiley, Diana, and Bortz, Walter M., II. "Sexuality and Aging—Usual and Successful," *Journals of Gerontology,* May 1996, pp. M142-M146.

Willett, Walter C., et al. "Mediterranean Diet Pyramid: A Cultural Model for Healthy Eating," *American Journal of Clinical Nutrition,* June 1995, pp. 1402S-1406S.

Winger, Jean Merhinge, RN, MSN, NP-C. "Age Associated Changes in the Endocrine System," *Nursing Clinics of North America,* December 1996, pp. 827–843.

Wirth, Lori A., BA, MHSE. "Plotting the Food Pyramid: An Evaluation of Dietary Patterns," *Journal of School Health,* 1996, pp. 225–228.

Wise, David A. "Retirement Against the Demographic Trend: More Older People Living Longer, Working Less, and Saving Less," *Demography,* February 1997, pp. 83–85.

Zuber, Thomas J., MD. "Rosacea: Beyond the First Blush," *Hospital Practice,* February 15, 1997, pp. 188–189.

Index

reading, 179
Rehman, Jamil, 109
restless legs, 86
retinas, 92
retirement, 155–158, 160–161
retirement communities, 172–173
Riley, John Jr., 191
Riley, Matilda, 191
Rimm, Eric, 74, 75
risky behavior, 180–183
Ritter, Malcom, 93
Roenigk, Henry, 93
rosacea, 41–42
  laser surgery for, 92
  makeup for, 42
Rosen, Donald, 25
Russell, Robert, 75

salt
  ability to eliminate, 46
  as conditioned response to, 46
  hypertension and, 77
  reducing use of, 77–78
  using herbs and spices instead of, 78
saving, 155–156
  for kid's college, 156, 161–162
  for retirement, 155–156, 160–161
Schiavi, Raul, 109
Schow, Douglas, 108, 110
Schuett, Dawn, 113
Schulte, Brigid, 182
sclerotherapy, 94
senior discounts, 190–191
senior moments, 139
SeniorNet, 191
sense of self, 26–27
sexuality
  and aging, 100
  barriers to, 101–103
  erectile dysfunction, 108–109
  importance of public education of, 113
  impotency, 84
  improving, 111–112
  lack of healthy partner, 102, 103
  male menopause, 108
  male sexual dysfunction and, 109–111
  medication and, 103
  menopause and, 106–108
  sexual dysfunction and 105–106
  stress and, 111

Shay, Kenneth, 39
Sherman, Art, 115
Sherman, Florence, 115
Ship, Jonathan, 39
Shockman, Luke, 62
Silverstein, Merril, 171
simplicity movement, 187
Simpson, Carol, 169
skin, 41–42, 46–47
skin cancer check, 70
Skoe, Eva, 125
sleep, 85–87
sleep deprivation, 86
Sloane, Philip, 48
slowing down, 178–180
smart aging tips, 32, 54, 68, 98, 116, 135, 154, 175, 194
Smith, Carol, 168
Smith, Lynn, 123
smoking
  Alzheimer's disease and, 146–147
  effects of, 95–96
  heart disease and, 45
  mental ability and, 145–146
  skin and, 41
  teeth and, 39
Snyderman, Nancy, 61
Social Security program, 155–156
Solomon, Renee, 18–19, 71, 96
soybeans, 47
speak out, 131
spices, 78
spicy foods, 47
spirituality
  benefits of, 29
  impact on health, 28–29
  importance of prayer/meditation, 188
  meditation, 174
  nature and, 29
spouse, loss of, 21, 102
Springer, Ilene, 87
Stamatiadis, Nikiforos, 36, 147
stamina, 51–52
Stanley, Thomas, 160
Stern, Ken, 171–172
Stevens, Joseph, 40
Stewart, Cynthia, 97
storytelling, family, 188–189
stress
  decreasing, 186–187
  identifying, 20–21

About the Author

Harriet Hodgson has been a nonfiction writer for more than 22 years. She has a BS degree in Early Childhood Education, with honors, from Wheelock College in Boston, and an MA in Art Education from the University of Minnesota in Minneapolis. After twelve years of teaching, she decided to change careers and turned to writing.

An experienced writer, Hodgson is the author of 20 books for parents and children, plus many newspaper and magazine articles. She is a contributing writer for *The Mayo Clinic Complete Book of Pregnancy and Baby's First Year*. She has also written Mayo Clinic resources to help young children and teens prepare for heart surgery.

She was both narrator and writer for "Parent Talk," broadcast on Minnesota Public Radio. A frequent radio and television guest, she has appeared on innumerable radio talk shows, including CBS and WCCO radio. She has also appeared on many television shows, including CNN. Hodgson is a freelance special features writer for the *Rochester Post-Bulletin*. Her children's books are detailed in the international library reference *Something About the Author*.

The mother of two grown daughters and the proud grandmother of twins, Hodgson lives in Rochester, Minnesota, with her husband, John.